UNLOCK the BENEFITS of CHAIR YOGA

This book is dedicated to my husband,
the biggest dreamer of all,
who refuses to give up!

Table of Contents

Chapter 8 123

Back Pain Relief Sequence 125

Achy Joint Sequence 130

Headaches, Migraines and Neck Tension Relief Sequence 138

Introduction

Yoga is one of the best self-care practices known to humanity. The moment you show an interest in your mental or spiritual health, yoga is guaranteed to be one of the first things recommended to you. You're sure to have relatives suggest it. Advertisements for yoga courses or yoga mats will surely pop up on your social media feeds. Yoga-centric YouTube channels will be on your recommended watch list.

This recommendation is not unfounded. Yoga is indeed one of the best things you can do for your mental, spiritual, and physical health. Yoga comes with a plethora of benefits that we will discuss in this book. It truly is worthy of all the hype.

However, not everyone is capable of downward dogging, of being a cobra or a crane, or even of sitting like a lotus. Yoga is a practice meant to increase flexibility and mobility. And, unfortunately, many who desperately need it don't have the flexibility or mobility to practice yoga.

Yoga is often depicted by young, fit, and healthy people simply improving their already healthy lifestyle. However, where yoga is needed most, it is often more difficult to achieve.

Consider someone who is recovering from a serious operation or medical treatment, someone who has had lifelong mobility issues and cannot walk, someone in a wheelchair, or one whose age is catching up with them in the form of arthritis, bad hips or knees, joint replacements, etc. Should those who need it most be denied the healing benefits of yoga?

Of course not.

"Chair pose is a defiance of spirit, showing how high you can reach when you're forced down." (Guillemets, 2002). Being forced down is no reason not to reach for the sky. Regardless of your mobility, yoga is accessible and available to you.

Yoga is not all about twisting yourself into a certain shape, or the most common comparison, twisting yourself into a pretzel. Yoga is not about being the most flexible and reaching each position with ease. Yoga is about showing up for your practice, listening to your body, accepting your abilities or their lack, pushing yourself, stretching yourself beyond what you are now and closer to what you wish to be. Yoga is about finding inner peace and strength.

You can do that without standing up. You can do that without buying a yoga mat and meditating in the first morning light in complete silence for an hour. You can achieve your goals in your desk chair or in your wheelchair. This book is going to help you do so. This book is going to give you the tools and knowledge to reach up, to reach for the sky, even if you feel forced down.

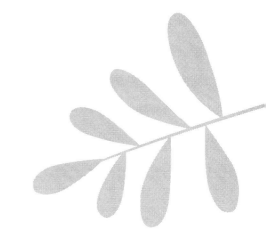

Chapter 1

THE EVOLUTION OF YOGA AND HOW IT REACHED THE WESTERN WORLD

It is widely known and understood that yoga originated in India. The most agreed upon origin of yoga dates back to the Vedic Period (4,500–1,200 BCE), although there is some evidence to suggest that it dates even further back, to the Indus Saraswati Valley in 2,700 BCE in ancient India.

However, even as far back as that, yoga started off with the three same basic principles it has today:

- Body postures and poses
- Breathing techniques
- Concentration and mental focus

The next known records of yoga are the Upanishad Texts (900–500 BCE), which introduced us to breathing control and mental concentration known as pranayama and pratyahara, respectively.

Thereafter, there are many texts that were found or published that changed and shaped yoga into what it is today. The Pali Canon (circa 600 BCE) described yogic poses and breathing exercises as well as the "Word of the Buddha." The Mahabharata (circa 400 BCE to 300 CE) is where clear reference is made to the three types of yoga:

- Yoga of Action: Karma Yoga
- Yoga of Devotion: Bhakti Yoga
- Yoga of Knowledge: Jnana Yoga

As the transportation of people and knowledge between countries and continents became easier, the ancient tradition of yoga spread beyond India. As it traveled through the world, the intent behind yoga was morphed. The rest of the world was introduced to the benefits of the practice.

Four main figures played a role in introducing yoga to the western and modern world: Tirumalai Krishnamacharya, Pattabhi Jois, BKS Iyengar, and Indra Devi. Based on the different intentions and the different teachings, yoga soon found itself being split up into separate yogic practices; some more focused on spiritual awakening and others more focused on physical health and bodily improvements.

Chapter 2

CLASSIC YOGA, MODERN YOGA, AND THE EIGHT LIMBS OF YOGA

The history of yoga up to this point is known as Pre-Classical Yoga. From 200 BCE to 500 CE marks the period known as Classical Yoga. This is when Patanjali's Yoga Sutras introduced the concept of hatha yoga (which we will discuss in the next chapter) as well as the theory of yoga.

And it's within Classical Yoga that the eight limbs of yoga are introduced. These eight limbs resemble the eightfold path of reaching the full benefits of yoga. They are:

- Yama
- Niyama
- Asana
- Pranayama
- Pratyahara
- Dharana
- Dhyana
- Samadhi

Yama

Yama is the first limb of eight. It refers to a moral code, or vows and disciplines regarding the world around us and how we interact with it. The point of Yamas is to ensure that you are benefitting in every facet of your life, not just the physical and mental. The goal is to ensure that you are strong and peaceful in your everyday life, not just while doing yoga.

The five Yamas are:

- Ahimsa: non-violence
- Aparigraha: non-greed
- Asteya: non-stealing
- Brahmacharya: correct use of energy
- Satya: truthfulness

Niyama

The prefix "ni" translated from Sanskrit means "within." Therefore, Niyama refers to actions directed towards ourselves as well as the world around us. The five Niyamas are:

- Ishvara Pranidhana: surrendering to a higher power
- Santosha: contentment
- Saucha: cleanliness
- Svadhyaya: self-reflection or self-study
- Tapas: discipline and burning desire

Asana

This is probably the most well-known and well-understood of the limbs: postures and poses. Asana actually means "seat," and should be steady and comfortable. These postures are meant to avoid distractions of pain and aches in the body and to find restfulness.

Pranayama

Pranayama is also a well-known limb of yoga: breathing techniques. The prefix "prana" means "energy" or "life source." The word pranayama can be interpreted in two different ways. Either as "prana-yama," meaning breath control or restraint; or as "prana-ayama," meaning freedom of breath.

Pratyahara

The prefix "pratya" means "withdraw" while the suffix "ahara" refers to taking things into ourselves through our senses (sight, hearing, smelling, touching, and tasting). Therefore, pratyahara refers to sensory withdrawal. Now, pratyahara doesn't refer to physically removing sensory stimulations. It rather means to focus so deeply on something that we are no longer bothered by external stimuli.

Dharana

Dharana is the sixth limb of eight, meaning "focused concentration." Dharana, pratyahara, and pranayama are all linked closely together and must often be done together in order to achieve the full effect. By practicing pratyahara and pranayama effectively, you can reach dharana: intent concentration.

Dhyana

Dhyana is the seventh limb of eight and refers to meditative absorption. Dhyana is less a practice than it is the result of effectively practicing the previous three limbs correctly. You may have done pratyahara, pranayama, and dharana and *feel* that you are meditating. Dhyana is an actual meditation.

Samadhi

Samadhi is the end goal of yoga: enlightenment or bliss. As with the other limbs, it is important to dissect the word further to gain a fuller understanding, for bliss may not mean what you think it does.

"Sama" refers to "equal" or "same." "Dhi" means "to see." In this meaning of the word, bliss does not refer to escapism and leaving our problems behind. Samadhi is *realization*; specifically, the realization of the life that lies ahead of us without any filters or disturbances.

✳ ✳ ✳

It's no secret that the yoga practiced today is not the same yoga that was practiced in ancient India. Of course, the core principles are generally the same, but the intention of people and the practice itself is very different—not only from what it used to be, but even from person to person.

For instance, for those in ancient India, the topmost priority when practicing yoga was to reach spiritual enlightenment and mental calmness. And while that is surely a great bonus for modern folk, the main focus nowadays is flexibility, strength, and physical improvement.

There are nine types of modern yoga practice:

- Hatha yoga: We cover hatha yoga in-depth in the next chapter.
- Vinyasa yoga: focuses on technique and poses in order to stretch and strengthen muscles.
- Bikram yoga (or hot yoga): Twenty-six standard poses that are practiced in an environment at a temperature of 35–40°C (95–104°F). The goal is to warm and stretch all the muscles and tendons of the body, as well as to detoxify and build endurance.
- Ashtanga yoga: focuses on the eight limbs of yoga—external and internal cleansing for the goal of the development of mental and spiritual health.
- Anusara yoga: focuses on improving flexibility, balance, and lung capacity. The goal is to feel relaxed and rejuvenated.
- Kundalini yoga: The main goal is spiritual healing and includes meditation, mantras, movement, poses, and breathing.
- Iyengar yoga: Refers to finding and practicing the perfect posture and then holding it for a period of time in an attempt to improve concentration, balance, and core strength.
- Sivananda yoga: There are twelve standard poses in this yoga practice, with the goal of fighting respiratory problems and psychological disorders. It includes improving one's lifestyle in an effort to minimize negative effects on the body.
- Yin yoga: focuses on strengthening the tendons and ligaments in the body. Similarly to Iyengar yoga, Yin yoga also involves holding practiced poses for a period of time.

Chapter 3

HATHA YOGA VERSUS CHAIR YOGA

Hatha Yoga

"Ha" refers to the esoteric sun and "tha" refers to the moon. Therefore, hatha yoga is a practice that aims to join and balance two energies. Hatha yoga involves breathing techniques and a set of postures that are held for a time before slowly moving into the next.

The literal definition of the word "hatha" is "force" and, using this definition, hatha yoga can be described as "the yoga of force." Most types of modern yoga are just variations and forms of hatha yoga. Originally, hatha yoga was practiced as a way to prepare the body for long periods of meditation. However, modern yoga has a different goal in mind than traditional yoga: fitness.

Traditional yoga was meant to be a spiritual experience, whereas modern yoga focuses more on the physical benefits. Of course, modern yoga can be made spiritual if the practitioner wishes for it. The main difference, however, is the asanas and other limbs of yoga are performed.

In fact, asanas were not a very important part of modern yoga when it first cropped up in the nineteenth century. The first wave of modern yoga was headed by a man named Swami Vivekananda who largely ignored and rejected hatha yoga and asanas as an important part of yoga. He focused more on pranayama and positive thinking. It was only later, in the 1920s, that asanas regained their importance in modern yoga and hatha yoga gained popularity.

Chair Yoga

As mentioned above, most of the modern yoga practiced nowadays is some variation of hatha yoga. Chair yoga is no different. Chair yoga is a modified variation of hatha yoga specifically for those who cannot perform standing yoga or yoga on the floor. Chair yoga is also a very beneficial practice for those looking for movement that will have a low impact on their joints.

Ultimately, chair yoga can be described as hatha yoga performed on a chair. Chair yoga consists of the seated poses of hatha yoga, as well as other poses of hatha yoga that have been modified to be performed in a seated position.

Chair yoga, much like "normal" yoga, comes with a plethora of benefits to those who practice it. Regularly practicing chair yoga may:

- improve blood circulation and oxygenation
- improve flexibility and mobility
- improve balance
- build strength
- improve breath control
- aid in pain management
- reduce blood pressure
- calm the nervous system
- reduce stress and depression
- aid in weight loss by burning calories and reducing the risks of overeating due to stress or depression
- promote independence and confidence
- improve mindset and outlook on life
- rejuvenate the soul
- improve mental focus

Why Should Seniors Practice Chair Yoga?

Chair yoga is an accessible, easy, and low-impact way of getting the body to move and stretch. Physical exercise and stretching of the muscles can slow or reduce the effects of aging on the bones, muscles, and joints. As we get older, our muscle mass naturally declines, our bones naturally become more fragile, and our joints lose lubrication and mobility. Regularly moving and stretching the muscles can help to slow these aging effects down significantly.

Chair yoga also builds strength in our aging muscles. Muscle growth improves balance, which reduces the risk of falling and injuring ourselves. It also lessens the pain that is associated with many age-related conditions like arthritis.

Chair Yoga Versus Chair Exercises

Chair yoga refers to practicing yoga while seated in a chair (or in a seated position). Chair yoga is a practice designed to be accessible for those with disabilities or limited mobility.

Chair exercises refer to exercises that are performed using a chair as a piece of equipment, such as chair squats, chair leg raises, etc.

While both chair yoga and chair exercises can improve flexibility and strength, only chair yoga focuses on incorporating mindfulness, breathing techniques, and relaxation.

Chapter 4

FAQS AND CONSIDERATIONS

FAQs

What is chair yoga? Simply put, chair yoga is practicing yoga while seated. Chair yoga focuses on asanas that can be performed while sitting down.

Why practice chair yoga? Accessibility. Asanas that require you to be on the ground or require you to be standing are not possible for all those who wish to gain the benefits of yoga. Practicing chair yoga properly can offer the benefits of yoga to those who arguably need it the most.

Who can benefit from chair yoga?

- The elderly
- Those who are:
    - recovering from surgery
    - going through or recovering from medical treatment
    - struggling with mobility issues
    - in wheelchairs
    - bedridden
    - struggling with mental/physical disorders that prevent them from standing up or going down onto the floor
    - struggling with situational/locational challenges that prevent them from standing up or going down onto the floor

Can I practice chair yoga if I have never done yoga before? Of course. Just as with traditional yoga, chair yoga comes in different levels of difficulty. You can start off with very easy poses and slowly build up. This book was made for beginners, but each sequence increases in difficulty. This means that there will be detailed step-by-step instructions on each asana, as well as detailed images for reference.

What kind of chair should I practice chair yoga on? The most important aspect of the chair should be its sturdiness. As long as the chair won't move around as you're doing the poses, it should be perfect.

Do I need any extra equipment to do chair yoga? No. You don't need a yoga mat or special yoga clothes. You should wear something comfortable and something that will allow you to move around easily. While no equipment is necessary, you can use foam blocks or light weights, and a strap of some kind can come in handy for the more difficult poses. You can use a mat or carpet to prevent your chair from moving around.

Can I practice chair yoga if I have high blood pressure? Yes. In fact, a review conducted by Wu et al. in 2019 showed that those who practiced yoga for an hour five times a week for thirteen weeks reported reductions in their blood pressure. While there are some asanas to avoid if you have high blood pressure, many of them are floor poses.

Can I practice chair yoga if I have significantly limited mobility? Chair yoga is a practice of yoga that is highly accessible to those with mobility issues. There may still be poses or stretches that prove more difficult. However, this book contains many different variations for different intensities. The goal is to get your body moving, not to reach the highest difficulty level in the first sitting.

Can I practice chair yoga if I have problems with balance? You may find certain poses and stretches to be more difficult, even while seated. It's important to only practice chair yoga at a level where you feel comfortable and safe. Over time, and with regular practice, your balance will improve.

Can I practice chair yoga if I have joint pains? You can practice chair yoga with joint pains. However, some poses may be much more painful than others. The important thing is to get started and observe your body.

Can I practice chair yoga if I have bad flexibility? Of course. The point of yoga is to slowly stretch the muscles, not to force yourself into certain shapes just for the sake of it. Yoga is beyond flexibility; it's about breathing, about controlling the mind, and about consistency to achieve your goals.

What if I struggle to follow the instructions for chair yoga? It is common for some people to find it more of a challenge to comprehend the directions for certain poses and stretches. This can lead to frustration, incorrect form, or significant difficulty. It's important to take this book one chapter at a time. Focus fully on getting the hang of each breathing exercise, and each pose, before moving on to the next. Perfecting one pose may help you more easily go into the next.

Is there such a thing as overdoing yoga? Absolutely. Just as with any other physical activity, it is extremely important to moderate yourself and not push your body beyond its limits. Doing so will only undo all the benefits of practicing yoga in the first place. Eve Chalicha from the BetterMe blog recommends practicing yoga two or three times a week and giving your body time to recover between sessions. Of course, you can practice yoga more regularly, but you should practice it at a lower intensity—no more than ten to twenty minutes per day. It's important to let your muscles rest as well.

Can I practice breathing exercises every day? Yes, you can. That would be very beneficial, as it would help you relax and improve your overall well-being. Also, it would help in your chair yoga practice.

Will chair yoga improve my core strength? If practiced consistently, absolutely.

Will chair yoga improve my balance? If practiced consistently, absolutely.

Can I practice chair yoga at home, or should I go to a studio? You can practice chair yoga in your own comfortable environment. The point of chair yoga is accessibility and convenience. Therefore, you should practice chair yoga wherever you are able and are comfortable doing so.

Can I practice chair yoga if I have back pains? Of course. Some poses may prove more painful or difficult, but this book has exercises included for those with back pain.

Considerations

If you are concerned about injuring yourself by practicing chair yoga, the best course of action is to talk to your doctor or physical therapist. Show them the asanas (poses) you plan to practice and ask them to recommend postures that are suitable for your health condition.

It's important to remember that yogic postures are eased into slowly and there is a heightened focus on the body. If you feel pain, do not push yourself farther. If you are struggling to ease into an asana, try one of the variations. If none of the variations are working, skip that asana and move on to the next. You should never be in pain while practicing.

Another important aspect of being comfortable while in asanas is remembering to breathe. You should not be holding your breath while in an asana unless directed to do so—and even when directed to do so, it should never be longer than a couple of seconds. This is why it would be beneficial to practice breathing exercise every day.

Important things to remember while practicing chair yoga (or yoga of any kind):

- Consistency is the key to achieving your goals. Practice regularly. You will not achieve any results by practicing once every other week.
- You don't have to have the perfect form. Follow the directions to the best of your ability and only to a point where you are comfortable.
- Yoga is not a competition or a race. Work at your own pace and use the variations that work best for you.
- Pay special attention to your head and neck alignment to avoid any pain.
- Those with **spinal disc problems** or **glaucoma** should take special care to choose postures that do not involve any twists or inversions.
- It is better not to have a big meal before practicing chair yoga.
- Remember to do the warm-up exercises before practicing chair yoga. Warm muscles are capable of stretching farther without strain.

Chapter 5

PRANAYAMA
(BREATHING EXERCISES)

Breathing is a critically important facet of yoga and chair yoga alike. Pranayama is one of the eight limbs of yoga, which must be mastered in order to master the other limbs as well. Here is why breathing is so important when practicing yoga:

- Focusing on breathing offers the body more oxygen through muscle contractions and releases. This allows your muscles to perform at a greater capacity.

- Breathing helps you get into the mindful and concentrated state needed to achieve dharana and samadhi.

- Ujjayi breathing (discussed later in this chapter) regulates the internal heat of the body, cleansing the system, protecting your organs during stretching, and improving your ability to hold postures.

- Breathing exercises put you in the right emotional and mental state to be calm and enjoy the peacefulness of yoga.

Beyond this, learning effective breathing techniques offers many benefits in and of itself.

- Reduces stress: Pranayama calms the nervous system.

- Improves mindfulness: By focusing your energy on something, usually an automatic function of the body, you are also practicing your ability to focus on the present and on your body.

- Improves lung function: Because breathing is automatic, it is not often that we practice and strengthen it. However, learning to improve your breathing techniques teaches your lungs to literally get better at breathing.

- Improves quality of sleep: The benefits of proper breathing techniques lead to an improved quality of sleep, as you are able to find rest sooner and breathe easier in your sleep.

- Reduces high blood pressure: Learning to control your nervous system may help in minimizing the risk of hypertension.

- Improves cognitive performance: The combination of learned control of the nervous system, focus, and mindfulness improves the brain's overall cognitive performance. This leads to enhanced executive function, auditory memory, and sensory-motor performance.

✿ Reduces cravings for cigarettes: Studies have shown (Nunez, 2020) that regular yogic breathing exercises reduced the cravings, as well as the negative effects of withdrawal, in those trying to quit smoking.

Now, when I say breathing techniques, I don't simply mean inhaling to the count of three and then exhaling to the count of three. I don't simply mean breathing in through the nose and breathing out through the mouth. There are many different breathing techniques out there.

We will discuss a few here. All of these breathing exercises should be practiced for three to five minutes spread throughout the day. As you grow more comfortable with these practices, you can increase the duration of your practice.

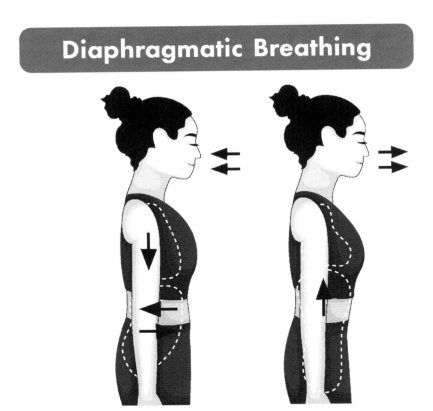

Diaphragmatic breathing refers to belly or abdominal breathing. The technique goes as follows:

✿ Ensure that you are sitting, relaxed and in a comfortable position, with your knees bent.

- Place one hand on your upper chest and place the other below your ribcage. You should be able to feel the movement of your diaphragm as you breathe.

- Breathe in slowly and deeply through your nose so that your stomach presses against your hand.

- Do your best not to let your upper chest press against the hand you have placed there.

- Exhale through puckered lips and engage your abdominal muscles, also without letting your upper chest press against your hand there.

The goal with diaphragmatic breathing is to breathe air into the belly, using your diagram, rather than simply bringing air into the lungs. When you fill your lungs with air, your chest will rise and fall and effectively press against the hand you have resting on it. The goal is to keep the hand on your upper chest as still as possible, and only have the hand on your stomach move up and down as you breathe.

The benefits that come with diaphragmatic breathing are:

- decreased muscle tension
- reduced heart rate and blood pressure
- improved blood oxygenation
- improved concentration
- increased energy and motivation
- increased warmth of your hands and feet
- strengthened immune system
- reduced stress hormones
- reversed stress response

Dirga Pranayama

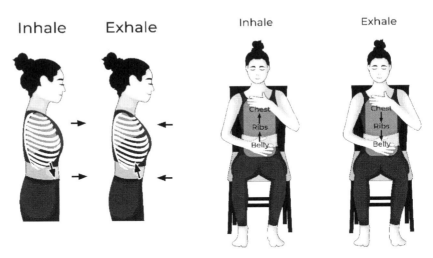

Inhale Exhale Inhale Exhale

Dirga pranayama, or three-part breathing, refers to focusing your breath on three parts of your torso: the lower belly, the lower chest, and the lower throat. The technique goes as follows:

- This breathing technique can be practiced either lying flat on your back or sitting comfortably in a chair. Be sure that your chest is open and your body is relaxed. It's preferred that you sit cross-legged, but it is not necessary. It's fine if you're sitting on the chair with feet flat on the floor.

- Each breath should be inhaled and exhaled through the nose, slowly.

- The goal of this breathing exercise is to eventually inhale and allow the breath to move from your lower belly, to your lower chest, and then to your lower throat. When you exhale, it should start in the lower throat, then move to your lower chest, and then to your lower belly.

- When beginning this breathing exercise, you may place your hands on these parts of your body to feel the air expanding and contracting the area.

- Start first by inhaling air into the belly and letting it expand with each inhale, and flatten with each exhale. Do this until you are comfortable with the motion.

- Next, take in a deep belly breath and when your belly is expanded, draw in another small breath and focus it into the chest. You should move your hand up to your lower chest and feel it expand.

- When exhaling, first expel the air in your chest and then the air in your belly, allowing both to deflate fully. Do this until you are comfortable with the motion.

- Next, breathe into the belly, then into the lower chest, and then draw in one last breath to fill the upper chest up to the collarbone. Your entire chest should expand fully.

- When exhaling, first expel the air in your upper chest, then the air in your lower chest, and then the air in your belly. Let each part deflate before moving on to the next.

The benefits that come with dirga pranayama are as follows:

- Aids in oxygenating the blood
- It is a useful relaxation technique to deepen your breath
- Increased blood flow promotes improved focus

Ujjayi Pranayama

Ujjayi (victorious or ocean) breathing refers to prolonged, controlled, and deep breathing. The technique goes as follows:

- Sit comfortably with your back straight and your shoulders relaxed.
- Each breath should be inhaled and exhaled through the mouth.

- On each exhale, pretend that you are using your breath to fog up a pair of glasses. Constrict your soft palate so that you hear a soft hissing noise on each exhale. Do this until you are comfortable with the motion.

- Then, apply the same technique to your inhaled breaths. You should continue hearing the soft hissing noise as you constrict your soft palate on the inhale. Do this until you are comfortable with the motion.

- When you are comfortable with this breathing technique, slowly shift to breathing through your nose. Close your mouth and breathe through the nose while still applying the same control to your throat.

- Each breath should be slow, long, and deep.

The benefits that come with ujjayi breathing are as follows:

- Increases oxygen consumption

- Promotes relaxation by calming the nervous system's stress response

- Strengthens the power and direction of your breath, allowing you to direct your breath into parts of the body that need it during your yoga sessions

Bhramari Breathing

Bhramari (bee or humming) breathing is a very easy breathing technique that is dedicated to building a relationship between breath and emotional state. The technique goes as follows:

- Sit in a comfortable position with your back straight and your shoulders stretched.

- Type 1 bhramari breathing:
  - Breathe deeply and slowly through the nose.
  - On each slow exhale, make a deep and steady humming noise.

- Type 2 bhramari breathing:
  - Breathe deeply and slowly through the nose.
  - Bring your hands to your face. Place your

  - thumbs against each tragus (the bump at the very front of your ear canal)
  - index fingers against the inner corners of your eyes
  - middle fingers against the sides of the nose
  - ring fingers above the lips
  - pinky fingers below the lips
- Apply light pressure to the eyeballs.
- On each slow exhale, make a deep and steady humming noise.

The benefits of bhramari breathing are as follows:

- Relieves stress by promoting the healing capacity of the body
- Improves blood circulation
- May help with hearing conditions
- Aids in emotional regulation

Nadi Shodhana Breathing

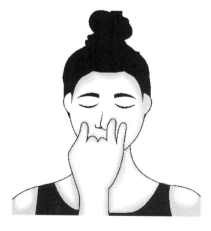

Nadi shodhana, or alternate nostril breathing, is exactly as it sounds: breath control through breathing through alternating nostrils. The technique goes as follows:

- Sit in a comfortable position.
- Each breath will be inhaled and exhaled through the nose.
- Bring your hand up to your nose, resting your thumb and ring finger on either side of your nose lightly, without closing your nostrils.
- First, press your thumb against your right nostril, closing it. Exhale slowly and fully through your left nostril.
- Release your right nostril and press your ring finger against your left nostril, closing it. Inhale slowly and deeply.
- Release your left nostril and press your thumb back down on your right nostril.
- Repeat this process throughout the breathing exercise.

The benefits of nadi shodhana breathing are as follows:

- Reduces stress by regulating the nervous system
- Reduces blood pressure

Sama Vritti Pranayama

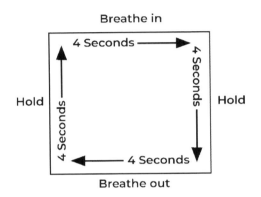

Breathe in

4 Seconds

4 Seconds

Hold

4 Seconds

Hold

4 Seconds

Breathe out

Sama vritti pranayama is also known as "box" and "equal" breathing. Sama Vritti breathing is ratioed breathing that uses a set length of inhalation, breath holds, and exhalations. The technique goes as follows:

- Sit in a comfortable position.
- Each breath will be inhaled and exhaled through the nose.
- At your own comfortable pace, start to slow and deepen your breathing to a point where you are still breathing easily and without losing your breath.

- The breath cycle for sama vritti is:
  - Inhale for four seconds.
  - Hold the breath for four seconds.
  - Exhale for four seconds.
  - Hold the breath out for four seconds.

The benefits of sama vritti pranayama are as follows:

- Reduces mental anxiety
- Slows your heart rate
- Increases oxygenation of the brain
- Improves focus

Chapter 6

TWO WARM-UP SEQUENCES

Before jumping into practicing chair yoga, it is important to first warm up your muscles. There are four reasons to never skip warm-up exercises. Warm-up exercises:

- **Prepare the body.** By spending just five to ten minutes warming up, you increase the blood flow to your muscles by 75 percent, which improves their strength and flexibility.

- **Reduce any risk of injuries.** By increasing the blood flow to your muscles, they are able to stretch farther without undergoing excessive strain.

- **Prepare the mind.** Your warm-up exercises can serve as the transition from busy, everyday life into the calm and relaxed state of practicing yoga. You can use your warm-up practice to still your mind, focus your breathing, and find a comfortable seating position that will work for the whole session.

- **Optimize poses and performance.** If your muscles are able to bend farther, you will be able to ease into poses more easily and hold them without pain or discomfort. If you are less concerned about hurting yourself, you can focus more deeply on stilling your mind and on your breathing. If you are fully in the mindset, you can achieve greater results.

If you're entirely new to chair yoga practice, you can start practicing by choosing one of the breathing exercises and adding one of the warm-up sequences from chapter 6.

This way, you will familiarize yourself with the way the practice flows.

The next time you can work on a different warm-up sequence combined with another breathing exercise.

These two warm-up sequences can be performed as a stand-alone practice or combined with one of the chapter's seven flows.

One more thing before we will move on to practice:

Before doing each asana, remember quickly to go through check-up points of your body position. Unless requested otherwise, when practicing chair yoga, most asanas will start in sitting up straight position with feet placed firmly on the ground. Think that you're lifting your heart to the sky.

Keep shoulders relaxed and the neck long. Don't be too tense, but at the same time don't be sluggish. Find the balance, feel your core being active. Don't rush; coordinate breathing with movement. Don't hold your breath unless the pose requires it. Remember to observe your face—smile. If you feel a strain in some part of the body, release the pose, return to the center, take a deep breath, and start again.

Your body and mind will become more flexible each time you practice.

Be consistent, make time, and show up for your practice—this is the most challenging part. I know that you can do it.

A Chair Yoga Warm-Up for New Beginnings

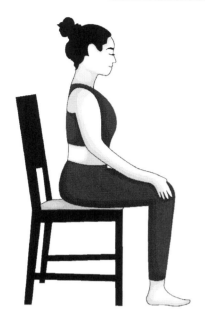

Chair Mountain Pose (Chair Tadasana). "Tada" means mountain and "asana" means a "pose."

Despite being a primary seated position that could also be performed in standing yoga, tadasana has many benefits. This is one of the foundational poses (asanas) in yoga, the same as diaphragmatic (deep or belly) breathing for breathing (pranayama) practice. Tadasana keeps your body actively aligned, which requires a certain level of body awareness.

Sit comfortably in the middle of the chair. Leave some space between the back of the chair and your back. Rock forward and back to find the seat bones. Feet flat on the floor, hip-distance apart. If you prefer, bring your knees together.

Start connecting to your breath.

Feel the connection between your feet and the floor.

If your feet are not resting on the ground, consider putting down a cushion, a folded towel, or a blanket to support your feet.

You can support the back with a bolster to keep the spine comfortable.

Press the feet firmly on the floor and extend the spine. Sit up straight, imagine that you have a crown on your head, and lift your chin slightly up. Take a deep breath in and out. Notice your breath. Lengthen the spine by exerting energy through the top of the head and down through sit bones.

Soften your shoulders, tongue, and eyebrows, and smile.

Close your eyes or soften your gaze, place your hands on your knees, and stay relaxed, breathing slowly and deeply. If your hands on your knees feel uncomfortable, keep them on your thighs with palms facing up or down.

Press the feet firmly on the floor and extend the spine to get comfortable.

Feel your feet flat on the floor and feel your heels and toes.

Remember to breathe. Be conscious.

Exhale to press your right foot firmly to the floor.

Inhale to release and relax the foot. Repeat—four to eight times for each foot.

Keeping that active feeling, move up to ensure your head is stacked over your heart, heart over your hips.

Before moving on to the Three-Part Breath pose, think of one thing you're grateful for and smile.

Three-Part Breath (Dirgha Pranayama)

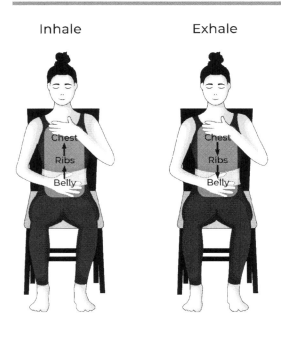

Inhale   Exhale

Three-part breath helps boost body energy and is usually performed as a warm-up exercise.

Sit up straight, stack your head over your heart, and your heart over your hips. Place your knees over your ankles and feel your feet planted firmly on the ground. Take a couple of deep breaths. Notice how your weight is distributed. Are you leaning more toward the left or right?

Feel your feet pressing gently onto the floor. The knees can be together or hip-distance apart. Try both ways and see which way feels more comfortable today. Tomorrow you could feel differently. Concentrate on what feels best right now.

Rest your arms on your thighs or knees.

You can place your right hand on the belly and your left hand on the heart. This will help you to feel and guide your breathing.

Start breathing into the belly. Feel how your belly and rib cage expand. Chest rises.

Exhale thinking that first, air leaves your chest, then your rib cage, and feel how your belly softens.

Repeat this for five to ten breaths. If you want to set the intention of the day, do so now.

Inhale: Belly – Ribs – Chest

Exhale: Chest – Ribs – Belly

If you're feeling dizzy, return to your normal breath.

Chair Neck Rolls

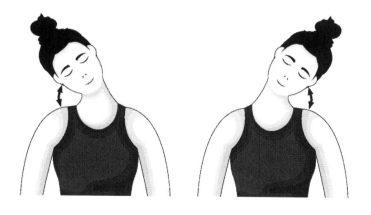

Chair neck rolls help to strengthen the neck, shoulders, and upper back.

People recovering from an accident, injury, or surgery could benefit from practicing neck rolls, which can speed up the recovery. Extending, bending and rotating the neck regularly can help maintain a normal range of motion. Chair neck rolls are targeted at the joint called atlas just below the skull that uses deep neck flexor muscles to facilitate movement and reduce tension.

These movements can work wonders on the nervous system when coordinated with breathing.

Sit tall and straight with your head stacked over your heart and your heart over your hips. Feel your feet firmly placed on the ground, hip-distance apart. Leave some space between your and the chair's back.

Rest your arms on the knees or thighs with palms facing up or down.

Take a couple of deep breaths.

Inhale and move your ear towards the right shoulder and exhale.

On the inhale, come back to the center, exhale, and pause before switching sides.

Repeat on another side: inhale, move your ear towards the left shoulder, relax, and exhale. Then inhale and return to the center.

Note: keep your shoulders relaxed; don't try to lift your shoulder to the ear. You bend your neck as far as your body allows today. With practice, your body's flexibility will improve. Concentrate on coordinating your movement with breath rather than how far you can reach.

Repeat this movement from neck/ear to shoulders while coordinating breath and movement. You can close your eyes if you like, and keep the body still yet relaxed.

Return to the center and pause with your breath before moving on to the next neck movement. Repeat the movement three to five times on each side.

Remember to breathe deeply.

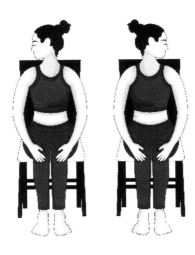

Rotating the neck will help to release the tension built around the neck and the shoulders. Stiffness around the neck and shoulders could cause headaches that could lead to a lack of sleep.

Come back to chair tadasana (mountain) pose.

Center and relax for a few breaths.

If you feel discomfort in the head due to movement of the neck, take deep breaths through both nostrils.

Inhale and lengthen through your spine. Ground down through the sit bones and imagine how the crown on your head rises towards the ceiling.

Tuck your chin in slightly.

Inhale and move your head to the right and exhale.

On the inhale, come back to the center, exhale, and pause before switching sides.

Repeat on another side: inhale, move your head to the left, relax, and exhale. Then inhale and return to the center.

Repeat two to four times for each side.

Chair Cat-Cow Pose (Chair Marjaryasana Bitilasana)

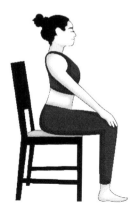

Chair Cat-Cow Pose is an effective way to tackle back pain, along with neck and shoulder stiffness. This therapeutic practice boosts flexibility as it stretches and massages the abdominal cavity, helping to improve digestion. Additionally, it increases the oxygenated blood supply in the spine, allowing a smoother and less painful movement of the back and neck muscles. Those with rheumatoid

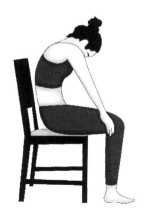

arthritis or osteoarthritis can benefit from this pose as the regular practice may help prevent these conditions from developing and reduce their symptoms at early stages. Opening and stretching these muscles and joints will help to support the entire pelvic girdle, thereby supporting the minor movements of the hips while walking, sitting, and lying down.

Note: If you have a neck, shoulder, spine, or hip injury, or have had recent abdominal surgery, you should avoid practicing the cat-cow pose and check with the doctor first.

Also, please **do not round** your spine if you have osteopenia or osteoporosis. On your exhale—return to a **neutral spine** instead of rounding.

Sit in a mountain pose. Relax and connect to your breath. Sit up tall. Feel a crown on your head rising towards the ceiling. Connect to your breath and take a couple of deep breaths. Rest your feet on the floor and keep your knees aligned with your hips.

Put your arms on your knees.

On the inhale, expand your chest. Let your head and chin go slightly back.

On the exhale, round your spine by curling the chest in.

Check if your shoulders are relaxed. Feel the space between your shoulders and earlobes. Keep breathing.

Practice coordinating your breath with movement. Don't rush. Smile, inhale, and repeat the movement three to five times.

Seated Pelvic Tilt Tuck

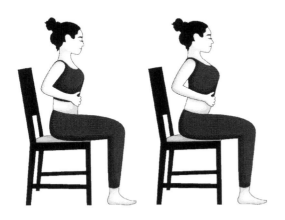

The practice of Seated Pelvic Tilt Tuck helps to build awareness of the various muscles that are engaged with the practice. The effective use of the abdominal muscles and the lower back muscles while they contract also builds deeper body awareness.

Place feet firmly on the floor in mountain pose, arms resting on your knees, spine erect.

Place your hands on top of the pelvis crest to feel the movement.

This is a slight movement, just tilting the tailbone back and forth.

Inhale as you tilt the pelvis forward, like tipping a bowl full of water ahead.

Exhale as you tilt the pelvis backward.

Repeat for six to eight cycles.

Practice on coordinating movement and breath.

Remember to keep your spine straight.

Chair Flexing Foot Pose

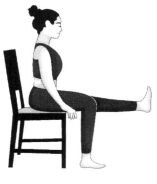

The Chair Flexing Foot Pose is a safe practice for students who have worn and torn ligaments at the knees and ankles, are healing from Achilles tendonitis, or are recovering from leg injuries or surgeries. A variation of this pose can also be performed lying in bed. During this movement, nerve cells in the joints are activated, resulting in better joint mobility and a better range of motion. This makes one's day-to-day activities easier to complete.

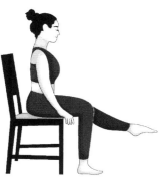

This is a great movement to increase blood flow to the lower extremities of the body, which can aid in reducing leg lymphedema, varicose veins, and other possible discomforts in the calves and feet.

Draw the crown of your head towards the sky and lengthen your spine. Place your hands gently on your knees. Start movement in mountain pose (Tadasana).

Begin by lifting the right leg and pointing the toes away from you.

Inhale, lift your toes towards your face, and press the heel away.

Exhale and point out the toes. Repeat a couple of rounds before switching the legs.

Repeat the left side.

Repeat each leg four to six times.

Easy Pose Chair One Leg Raised

Sukhasana Chair Urdhva Eka Pada

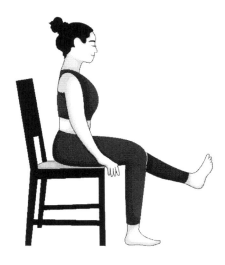

This move will help to stretch the ankles, soles, calves, and the back of the knees.

Sit up comfortably straight and relax your breathing. Check if both feet are flat and you can feel your toes, soles, and heels resting on the floor.

Keep your abdominals engaged.

On the inhale, raise the right leg parallel to the floor. Bring the toes upright and pull slightly towards yourself to feel the stretch. Try to keep the leg straight. Your left leg is firmly on the floor. Press through the heel of your foot. Stay centered and breathe deeply. Tighten the knees and the quads. See if you can stay there for several breaths. Repeat five times for each leg.

After you will complete the movement, put both feet on the ground and sit in a Tadasana.

Please take a couple of deep breaths and check how your body feels. Let your breath flow naturally. Close your eyes or soften your gaze. Sit for a couple of minutes, concentrating on your breath.

Finish the warm-up when your feel ready to move on.

Warm Up Your Mind and Body

Chair Mountain Pose

Chair Tadasana

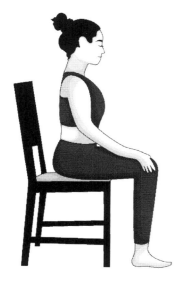

Sit comfortably in the middle of the chair. Leave some space between the back of the chair and your back.

Rock forward and back to find the sit bones.

Feet flat on the floor, hip-distance apart. Feel your feet-to-floor connection. If you prefer, bring your knees together. Start drawing energy from the ground through your heels and legs.

Stack your head over your heart and heart over your pelvis.

Start connecting to your breath.

Take a couple of deep breaths.

Sit straight but with no tension in your body. Check if you are hunching, if your neck feels long, if the shoulders are resting, the chin is slightly tucked in.

Breathe in and out. Connect to your deep breath. Feel your rib cage and belly expanding. Slowly breathe it out.

Repeat for a couple of rounds.

Chair Neck Stretch

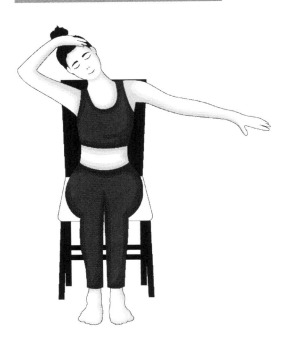

You will improve flexibility, mobility, and range of motion by practicing neck stretches. It also helps to reduce tension and stiffness in the neck.

Sit comfortably in the middle of the chair. Leave some space behind you. Don't lean on it.

Knees are stacked over your ankles, forming 90 degrees between your knees and hip.

Breathe in, and on your breath out, tilt your head towards your right shoulder, and place your right hand gently on the left ear. Extend your left arm. Stay in the pose and take a couple of deep breaths. You can breathe out with a slightly opened mouth.

Breathe in through your nose and return to the center with hands lying on your knees or thighs.

On the breath out, tilt your head towards your left shoulder, and place your left hand gently on the right ear. Extend your right arm. Stay there and take two deep breaths.

Repeat another two times.

Neck U Rotation Close Up

Kantha U Paryaayakrama

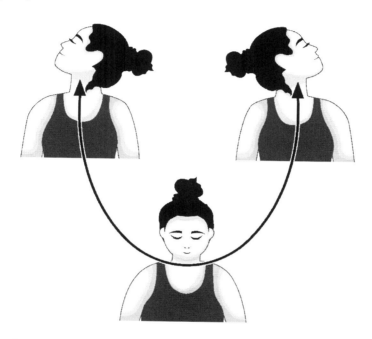

This stretches and strengthens the muscles around the neck and shoulders and the muscles in the upper back. The twist strengthens the side of the neck.

While the movement may seem simple, the improved range of motion helps with other poses and day-to-day activities.

Note: Avoid this pose if you have had any recent injury or surgery of the neck, shoulders, or upper back. Also, if you have acute spondylitis and extreme pain in the neck and shoulders or are experiencing an eye or ear infection, severe headache, migraine, vertigo, or dizziness, you should avoid this pose too.

Sit comfortably in the chair with a straight spine and feet on the floor. Let your arms rest at your sides. As you inhale, turn your head to the left, exhale, and tuck your chin towards your chest. Inhaling once more, move your chin toward the right shoulder, and exhale, rolling it back to your chest. Alternate between both sides until you return to a neutral position with the chin parallel to the floor. Stay here for two rounds.

Chair Seated Side Stretch Pose

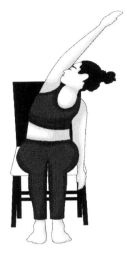

This pose is an opener for the shoulders and the neck. The arms are stretched to the opposite way. It is a great way to stretch. In addition to stretching, you increase awareness of your diaphragm and breathing.

Sit upright and keep knees hip-width apart or together. Place the hands on either side of the seat or your lap.

Roll your shoulders down the back.

Inhale, pulling in the core, sweep the right arm above the head, creating a lateral bend on the left-hand side. Exhale into the stretch. Allow your chest and head to tilt to the left. Stay in this pose for three breaths.

On the inhale, return to the center.

Repeat the same with the left side.

You can choose to stay on one side for two to three breaths before switching to the other side, or you may choose to move dynamically between one side and the other on the breath. Do what feels best for your body. During the movement, you may look down at the floor, straight ahead or up towards the top arm—please choose the option that feels right for your neck. Try to keep your mouth and jaw loose as you move.

Seated Cactus Arms Together Chair

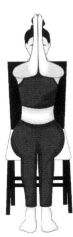

This pose is a simple shoulder movement called abduction of the shoulders. In this practice, the shoulders move away from each other, stretching the muscles completely. The range of motion can be increased by practicing cactus arms to ease and relax the upper body, especially your shoulders. This could also be beneficial for individuals recovering from a shoulder injury or surgery.

Inhale drawing your forearms towards each other in front of your face.

Allow your palms to touch and gently squeeze your elbows together. If your forearms cannot touch, don't worry about it. It's about bringing attention to the body and practicing movement and breath coordination.

Take five deep breaths and on the exhale release.

Chair Seated Twists

Chair Seated Twist is an effective exercise to stimulate the neck, hips and shoulders, while simultaneously engaging the muscles in one's back. The twisting action of the torso onto a grounded sit bone, combined with regular practice, helps to maintain mobility along one's spine. The chair provides excellent support, allowing one to easily remain in this twist while keeping their breath connected to their body movement. This practice can be used as a means of quickly releasing tension, energizing both body and mind.

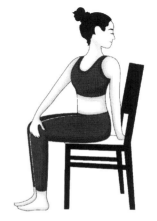

Note: If you're recovering after surgery to abdominal organs (like hernias, appendicitis, etc.), pelvic floor, or the lower back (like a slipped disc), you should consult a medical professional before practicing this pose.

Listen to your body. Don't perform a twist pose if your body feels uncomfortable, tense, or in pain. Take extra care when performing any twist poses.

Sit comfortably on the chair with shoulders relaxed.

Make sure you're not leaning on the back of the chair. Rock forward and back; find your sit bones. Sit tall with feet touching the floor, knees hip-width apart.

Inhale and place your arms over your head—lift and lengthen.

With the exhalation, twist left from the base of the spine. Your ribcage, shoulders, neck, and eyes go to the left, but the hips remain on the chair.

The right hand goes to the left knee, and the left hand is behind the left hip or on the back of the chair.

Breathe and feel the air filling up your body, and lengthen.

Exhale, continue to twist until you find your edge, and hold there. Check your knees to see if they're still in line with each other, that one is not ahead of the other.

Take a couple of deep breaths. Keep your shoulders away from your ears.

Chair Flexing Foot Pose

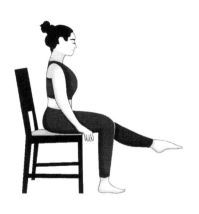

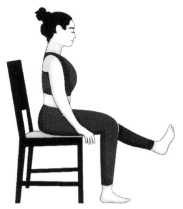

The Chair Flexing Foot Pose is a safe practice if you have worn and torn ligaments at the knees and ankles, are healing from Achilles tendonitis, or are recovering from leg injuries or surgeries. A variation of this pose can also be performed lying in bed. During this movement, nerve cells in the joints are activated, resulting in better joint mobility and a better range of motion. This makes one's day-to-day activities easier to complete.

Draw the crown of your head towards the sky and lengthen your spine. Place your hands gently on your knees.

Begin by lifting the left leg and pointing the toes away from you.

Inhale, lift your toes towards your face, and press the right heel away.

Exhale and point out the toes. Repeat a couple of rounds before switching the legs.

Repeat on the right side.

Repeat each leg four to six times.

This is a great movement to increase blood flow to the lower extremities of the body, which can aid in reducing leg lymphedema, varicose veins, and other possible discomforts in the calves and feet.

Heel and Toe Raises

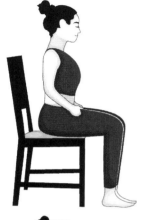

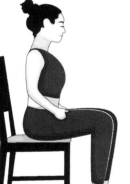

Sit nice and tall; roll the shoulders back.

Start with feet flat on the floor.

Inhale—lift both heels pressing the toes into the floor, and lower on the exhale.

Repeat five times.

Inhale—lift the right heel pressing the toes into the floor, and lower on the exhale.

Repeat five times.

Once the cycle is done, start lifting your toes.

Inhale—lift your right toes, pressing heels into the floor.

Exhale lower. Repeat the same with your left foot.

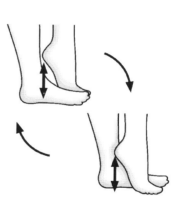

Repeat five times for each foot.

Lift the toes of both feet at the same time pressing the heels into the ground.

Repeat another three times.

Use your deep breath.

Ankle Crank on Chair

Goolf Ghoornan

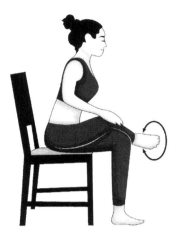

Sit nice and tall. Abdominals are engaged. Breathe in and imagine that you're lifting your heart up. Tuck your chin slightly in. Check if your upper body makes a nice angle with your hips, the same as the hips make a nice angle to your knees.

Both feet are pressing to the floor. Place right ankle on top of your left thigh.

Ensure the ankle is far enough over the thigh to be accessible for rotation.

Hold the right ankle with the right hand to support the ankle.

Hold the toes of the right foot if needed, with the left hand.

Using your hand or the ankle by itself, start to create circles with your foot.

Six to eight times clockwise, then six to eight counter-clockwise.

Repeat the same process with the opposite leg.

Chair Wide-Legged Seated Twist

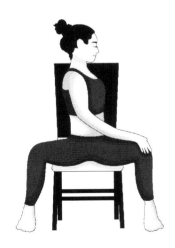

Wide-legged seated twist is very similar to the chair twist. Due to the position of the legs, this is a great hip opener. This pose brings a friendly and gentle stretch around the knees, lower back, and pelvic floor. Engaging the muscles of the pelvis, grounding, and twisting actions help maintain the correct posture, thus helping release the tightness in the neck, back, hips, and legs.

Note: It is not recommended for people who have undergone abdominal, pelvic floor, or lower back surgery, or who have been injured in the neck, shoulders, ribs, spine, hamstrings, or hip joints.

Sit nice and tall.

This time keep your knees wide at a comfortable width.

Inhale and sweep your arms above your head.

Exhale as you bring your right hand to your left knee.

Place your right hand on your left knee and keep your left hand behind you.

Inhale and start twisting to the left. Twist belly, ribs, chest, and head.

Stay there for a couple of deep breaths.

Inhale and come back to the center.

Repeat the same with the right side.

Do this two more times on each side.

Seated Corpse Pose

Savasana

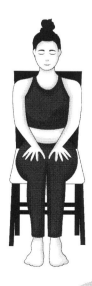

When you finish practice, sit with your eyes closed and your hands in your lap for a few minutes. Let your shoulders fall down and away from your ears. As you transition into the rest of your day, you will be able to absorb all the benefits of the poses you have done so far. Check how you feel. Breathe in through your nose and exhale through your mouth. Breathe in and feel the air traveling through your throat and to your belly. Open your mouth and exhale. Repeat for a couple of minutes.

Before you move to get on with your day, spend a few more minutes absorbing the good of your practice.

Observe your body without any judgment or effort. Pay attention to what's here in the present moment without needing to change anything. How does your body feel right now? Are there any physical sensations you are aware of? Notice the tightness or tension in specific parts and the ease or relaxation in others.

Breathe in, and by breathing out, release any tension in the body.

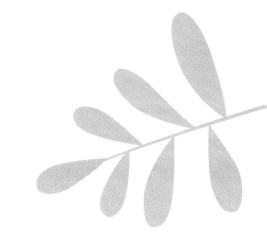

Chapter 7

This chapter has four sequences constructed with the progression in mind, as each sequence increases in difficulty.

To warm up your body, you can perform one of the sequences from chapter 6. However, this is optional, as every sequence in this chapter contains warm-up poses.

As mentioned, because the four sequences increase in difficulty gradually, I would recommend to start practice from the first.

Mountain Pose and Victorious Breath or Ocean Breath (Ujjayi)

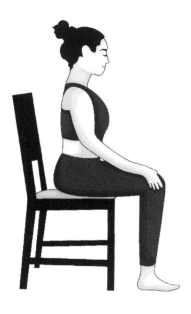

We talked about ocean breath in more detail in chapter 5. It's a beautiful breath as it energizes and calms the body simultaneously.

Aim to use it for this sequence. If you still are in the process of mastering it, don't worry; use your deep breathing technique and be mindful of coordinating breath and movement. Try to use when you can.

Let's begin in a mountain pose position.

Take a couple of deep breaths. Sit up nice and tall. Bring attention to your natural breath.

Check your neck and shoulders. Sit with your back straight and your shoulders relaxed. Roll your shoulders back. Keep your arms resting on your knees or your thighs with palms facing up or down.

Inhale through the nose, relax your jaw, and exhale through your mouth. When exhaling, you're almost creating a hhhaa sound. This breathing can also be described as a 'hissing' breath. You can also bring your hand towards your mouth and feel your warm breath. Breathe in, and when you breathe out, think that you intend to fog up the window. Once you have tried this a couple of times, breathe in through the nose, and on the exhale, we will keep the lips closed. The jaw will remain relaxed and bring your awareness to the back of your throat and make a slight restriction there.

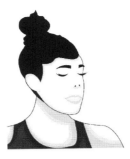 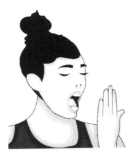

Practice this breathing for a couple of minutes. When you feel ready, move on the next pose.

Neck Side Stretch Pose

Warming up the neck will help to release the tension built around the neck and the shoulders. It also helps to reduce stiffness and increase the movement.

Sit up nice and tall. Bring attention to your natural breath.

Check your neck and shoulders. Sit with your back straight and your shoulders relaxed.

Roll your shoulders back.

Keep your arms resting on your knees or your thighs with palms facing up or down. Use ocean breath if it's available to you; if not, then be mindful with your breathing and coordinate breath with movement.

Inhale, and drop your shoulders down consciously, keeping the spine long. On the exhale, gently lower your left ear towards your left shoulder. Feel the stretch on the right side of the neck.

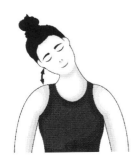

Inhale and come back to the center. Exhale, and drop your right ear towards your right shoulder.

Perform this movement five times on each side.

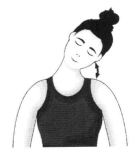

Neck Twists Head Down

Parivrtta Kantha Nata Sirsa

This exercise stretches and strengthens the shoulders and posterior muscles of the neck. These muscles allow the neck to twist and flex due to the neck and second rib movement. Furthermore, flexion neck rotation strengthens the sternocleidomastoid muscle (SCM), which is responsible for breathing, rotating the head from side to side, turning the neck, and bending the neck. Flexion neck strengthens the upper back muscles as well. A twist strengthens the side of the neck.

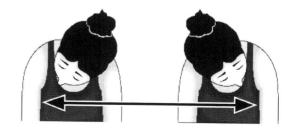

Note: The pose should be avoided if you have any recent injury or surgery of the neck, shoulders, or upper back.

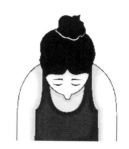

Keep sitting in Tadasana (mountain pose) with your back straight and arms rested on your knees.

Drop head to the chest.

Slowly and mindfully roll the head to one shoulder and hold for three to five breaths. Return to the center, keeping your chin tucked, and then roll to the next. Hold there for another three to five breaths.

Take your time. If you feel certain tight spots, stay there and breathe.

See if you can find more relaxation there.

Repeat three times on each side.

Shoulders Lift and Drop

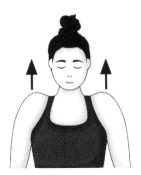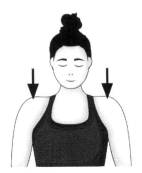

Our joints store a lot of stress and tension. While it is easy to act normal as we watch, read, and perform our daily activities, we are involuntarily creating many blocks around them. This emotional stress is loaded with a lot of pain and tension around the joints. By doing these shoulder lifts with mindful breathing, you can ease a lot of tension points.

Sit up tall and straight. Begin moving shoulders up as if you were trying to reach your earlobes. Inhale to raise the shoulders and exhale to drop the shoulders down.

Mindfully do this coordinated movement with your ocean breath five to eight times.

Chair Seated Shoulder Circles

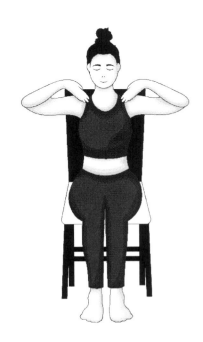

Warming up the shoulders and upper back with this pose can increase joint range of motion, flexibility, and strengthen the shoulders and arms.

Sit on the chair facing forwards, feet hip distance apart or together on the floor.

Inhale, lift your arms to the side, parallel to the floor. Exhale, and bring fingertips to shoulders.

Begin to circle in one direction. Circles can be large or small. Pause, and bring attention to your breathing.

Use your ocean breath and reverse the shoulder circles. Circle six to eight times in each direction.

Keep your spine straight.

Pause, inhale to open arms out, exhale lower arms down, and bring it to the center.

Arms To Side Rotations Chair

Parsva Hasta Paryayakrama

This exercise helps to strengthen the muscles of your arms and shoulders.

Sit. up tall and straight.

Raise your arms and spread them to the sides parallel to the floor, making a nice T.

Breathe in and start making small circles with your wrists in one direction. After a couple of breaths, make a few circles in the opposite direction.

If your arms feel tired, lower them onto your thighs on the exhale.

Take a few breaths in and out, and lift them to your sides again.

Start making small circles with your arms and slowly increase the motion, making them bigger, and then again, start rotating your arms in the opposite direction and making the circles small until you find stillness.

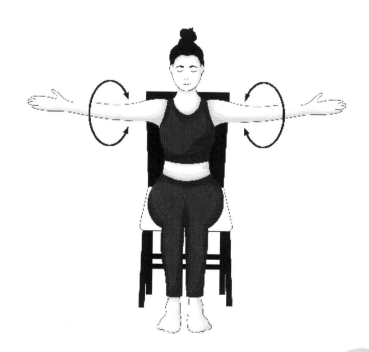

If your arms feel tired, lower them and gently shake them or sway them. Repeat the cycle when you feel ready.

Seated Cactus Arms Flow Chair

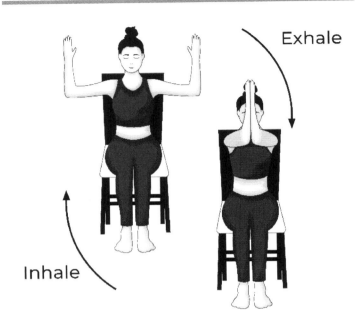

Exhale

Inhale

Moving the arms in and out enhances the lung capacity and develops strength in the diaphragm muscles. In this practice, the shoulders move away from each other, stretching the muscles completely. The range of motion can be increased by practicing cactus arms to ease and relax the upper body, especially your shoulders. This could also be beneficial for individuals recovering from a shoulder injury or surgery.

Draw the crown of your head towards the sky and lengthen your spine. Place your hands gently on your knees. Sit up nice and tall. Shoulders are relaxed; the spine is straight. Feel like you're grounding through the hips and feet.

Cactus arms, elbows in line with shoulders, wrists stacked over elbows. Spread the fingers and point them up. Breathe in and bring your arms to the side with your elbows bent as pictured.

Inhale and check if your core is active, the neck is long and, the shoulder blades are down the back.

Take a deep breath, lift through the chest, and squeeze the shoulder blades together. Listen to your body. As you exhale, bring your elbows, forearms, and hands together. Inhale, open your arms into a cactus position, and squeeze your shoulder blades together. Repeat the flow three to five times.

Work on coordinating the flow with the breath.

Chair Torso Circles

The exercise helps to strengthen the obliques, core, waist, and lower back.

Sit comfortably in the middle of the chair. Leave some space between the back of the chair and your back. Rock forward and back to find the sit bones. Feet flat on the floor, hip-distance apart or together.

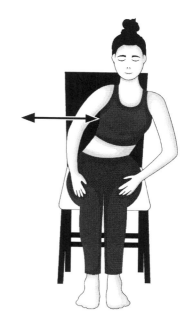

Feel your sit bones grounded to the chair.

Inhale as you roll your ribs forward.

Exhale and round your back.

Check that only the torso is moving. Legs should be firmly placed on the floor.

Draw big or small circles and listen to your body.

Repeat three to five times at your own breath pace. Use ocean or deep breaths.

Change direction, repeat.

Cobra Pose Chair

Bhujangasana

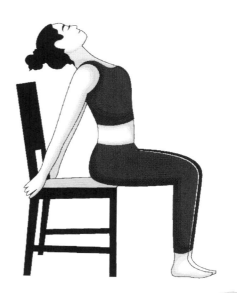

This pose strengthens your legs, upper back, lower back, shoulders, hamstrings, hips, glutes, and feet by engaging your legs, upper back, lower back, shoulders, hamstrings, hips, glutes, and feet. It can also help relieve stiffness in your shoulders, back, arms, and legs and elongate and lengthen your back.

Sit up nice and tall, closer to the edge of the chair, with your shoulders relaxed. Keep your knees together or hip-width apart.

Open your chest. Squeeze your shoulder blades together, look up, and bring your hands to the back of the chair.

Take the arms behind you on the inhale and hold on to the chair. Raise the chest and shoulders to look up. Your chin tilts upward and your eyes gaze toward the heavens.

Exhale, stay here in cobra pose chair feeling the stretch at the neck and upper chest.

Smile as you remain here for six breaths, breathing slow and deep. With each exhalation, feel the stretch.

Release, relax, and repeat to stay for the second round of six breaths.

If previous cobra pose is not available for you, try this variation.

Cobra Pose Chair Variation

As in all poses, sit up nice and tall, closer to the edge of the chair, with your shoulders relaxed. Keep your knees together or hip-width apart. Feet are flat on the floor.

Place your forearms on your thighs and keep your back as flat as possible.

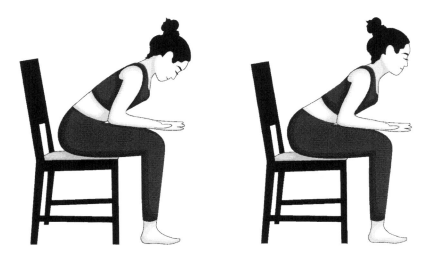

From this position, press on your hands, bring your chest forward and lengthen your spine as you keep your gaze on the ground.

Exhale, bending the torso over the thighs. Rest forearms on thighs.

Inhale as you lift your chest and head to look forward.

Exhale as you return your chest down toward your thighs.

Repeat slowly for several breaths.

Seated Twist Arms Shoulder Level Pose Chair

Upavistha Parivrtta Hasta Kandra

Twisting helps stretch out the spine. Gently rotating, this exercise loosens back muscles and all the fascia associated with them. It also encourages good health for tissues surrounding the spinal cord.

Begin by sitting on your sit bones on a chair you find comfortable.

Sit up nice and tall.

Keep some distance between the chair's backrest and your back. Let the back be straight and long, feet grounded, and ankles and knees in one straight line. Keep the feet together or apart.

Extend both arms to the sides in line with the shoulders, palms facing forward.

As you inhale, root the sit bones on the chair and lengthen the spine (imagine you are creating space between your vertebrae).

Exhale, twist to the right side originating from the lower back, taking the right hand to the back as far as possible and the left palm on the right shoulder.

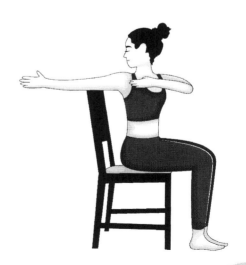

Keep your gaze on the right hand by gently and comfortably turning the neck.

Stay here for five deep breaths. Keep twisting slightly more with every exhalation (as much as possible without any strain) without moving the lower body.

With the next inhale, come back to the center, both arms open on the sides. Take a deep breath here.

Exhale, twist towards the left side originating from the waist, take the left hand to the back side and keep the right palm on the left shoulder.

Turn the neck gently to the left side and keep the gaze on the left hand. Make sure that the neck is not tense.

Feel the twist in the spine and a gentle stretch in the abdominal muscles, especially the obliques.

Stay here for five breaths.

Inhale, untwist to come back to the center, look in front, and release the hands down.

Seated Forward Bend Pose Chair

Paschimottanasana

The pose is a great stretch for the lower back and hamstrings.

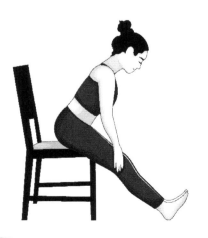

Note: People experiencing lower back or hamstrings injuries should take this practice slowly.

Sit closer to the edge of your chair (safely). Bring your legs out straight in front of you. Place your heels on the ground with your toes pointing out.

Breathe in, and check if your spine is straight. Lift your heart towards the sky.

Bend forward from the hips, keeping the spine elongated but don't round it on your exhale.

Keep legs straight but don't lock the knees. Have them slightly bent.

If you need to bend them more, just do it. Listen to your body. Your arms can hang at your side or you can put them on your legs but don't lean into them.

Hold for five breaths.

Feel how your hamstrings are stretching. If you need your hamstrings to stretch more, then pull your toes towards you.

Knee Head Down Chair

Anjaneyasana Variation Chair Uttana Hasta

Sit up nice and tall. Shoulders relaxed, and the neck is nice and tall. Feel as the crown on your head extends to the ceiling. Engage the core with your belly button pulled in. Don't lean on the chair.

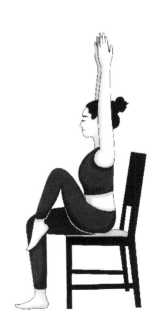

Roll your shoulder back. On the inhale, lift your arms and exhale.

Inhale and lift one knee and exhale to lower.

Repeat the same with the opposite knee.

Repeat six times on each side.

If your arms feel tired, lower them and let them hang next to the chair.

Inhale as you lift one knee up and exhale as you lower.

Repeat six times.

High Lunge Variation Chair

Ashta Chandrasana

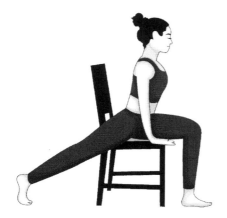

High lunge strengthens the quadriceps, gluteus maximus, calf muscles, and hamstrings. It also helps to improve balance and builds muscle to support the knee.

Sit nice and tall. Remember to breathe deeply. Use your ocean breath if you can.

Turn your body to the left with your left leg bent over the left side of the chair. The right leg is stretched out behind you to the right side of the chair, with your toes tucked. Your left hand can grab on to the side of the chair for support. Extend the spine upward, pulling the belly in and lifting the pelvic floor. Take three to four deep breaths.

If this pose feels too challenging, then bend your right leg slightly.

If you need a challenge, then on the inhale, reach the right arm towards the sky.

Exhale, release the arm down and turn the body to the front of the chair in tadasana (mountain pose), both feet flat on the ground.

Repeat on the right side.

Easy Pose Chair One Leg Opposite Arm Raised

Sukhasana Chair Urdhva Eka Pada Eka Hasta

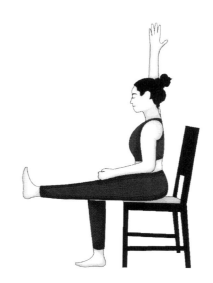

Sit nice and tall, away from the chair back. Use your ocean breath if you can.

Engage your core and pull the belly button in towards the spine.

Inhale and raise the right leg and left arm. Hold for a few breaths.

Feel how your leg is activated.

Lower the leg or bend through the knee if it's too challenging. Remember to breathe and coordinate movement with breath. Release to the ground after a couple of breaths.

Repeat two to three times for each side.

Mountain Pose

Tadasana

Sit comfortably in the middle of the chair. Leave some space between the back of the chair and your back. Rock forward and back to find the sit bones. Feet flat on the floor, hip-distance apart. If you prefer, bring your knees together.

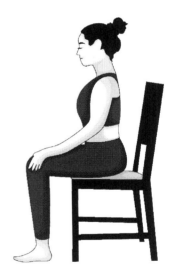

Draw your awareness towards the toes.

Inhale. As you pull the toes towards the body, try to spread all the toes with an equal distance between them.

Exhale as you bend the toes away from the body towards the floor.

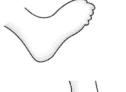

Think of one breath, one movement.

Repeat the practice, with the breath awareness in sync with the movement of the toes, for ten rounds.

Remain seated with your spine tall.

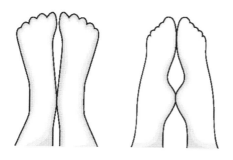

Move the soles of the feet inwards and outwards.

Allow the inner heels and toes to touch when you bring the feet inwards.

Repeat this movement with breath awareness—soles in and out for about ten times. Focus on the sync of the breath and movement. Keep sitting straight with shoulders relaxed.

Bee Breathing or the Humming Breath

Bhramari

Sit comfortably on the chair and maintain a straight spine. Rest your arms on your knees. Press your lips together and take a deep breath through your nose.

Make the sound "mmmm" as you exhale. Then repeat, breathe through your nose, and hum on the exhalation. Repeat for several minutes.

Once you finish, don't open your eyes and jump out of the chair. Sit quietly for a few more minutes. Ask yourself how your body feels.

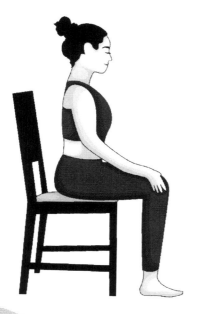

Smile, and thank yourself for turning up. Notice your thoughts but don't act on them. Let them go.

Or you can:

Place thumbs against each tragus (the bump at the very front of your ear canal).

Index fingers against the inner corners of your eyes and middle fingers against the sides of the nose. Place your ring fingers above the lips and your pinkies below the lips. On each slow exhale, make a deep and steady humming noise.

Sit and practice for a few minutes.

Check: how does your body feel? Is there any tension?

Be aware of the sounds which are surrounding you; can you smell anything? What is it? Can you recognize the smell? Don't try to keep thoughts away. Let them pass by and don't act on them. Observe the sounds around you; don't analyze them, simply listen. Thank yourself for turning up for your practice. Smile. Finish your routine when you feel ready.

Sequence Two
Chair Harmony and Strength

The Wings of Yoga
Lion's Breath (Simhasana)

Lion's breath can reduce stress, eliminate toxins, and stimulate your throat and upper chest. It is also known as lion pose in yoga. Lion's breath helps you clear your throat if you have a dry mouth or tickle in your throat. It also promotes relaxation in your facial and neck muscles, which helps when you've used them to talk or concentrate. Lion's breath may also help you release emotions, thoughts, or patterns.

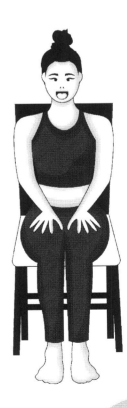

Sit comfortably on the chair and maintain a straight spine. You can lean on your chair backrest as long as you sit tall with your shoulders lowered.

Your hands can be put in a prayer position or on your knees. Lift your heart to the sky. Draw your attention to your natural breathing.

Unbend your arms and stretch out your fingers. This is to imitate a lion's claws. Inhale through the nostrils, then exhale with a loud "ha" from the mouth, extending your tongue as close to the chin as you can. While breathing out, focus on the middle of your forehead or the end of your nose. Fill up with breath and go back to neutral facial expression. Repeat four to six times.

Turtle Neck Flow to change the arrows

This movement lengthens and strengthens the neck muscles. The neck muscles are connected to the shoulders and back of the thoracic spine. This movement stretches those muscles.

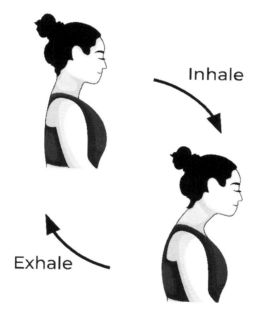

Note: If you have a neck and shoulder injury then skip this pose.

Sit comfortably on the chair and maintain a straight spine. You can lean on your chair backrest as long as you sit tall with your shoulders lowered. Keep your feet firmly on the ground.

On the inhale, take the chin forward, going beyond the chest and collarbone. Exhale to come back to the center.

Repeat it six times, making sure the extension is more with each round without moving the shoulders. Don't rush, as the slower you go, the better the sensation of the deeper stretch in tissues of the neck and shoulders.

Neck Stretch Variation

The same as the previous position, it will help you to warm up your neck muscles.

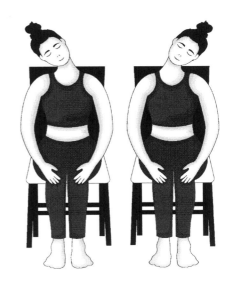

Sit comfortably in the middle of the chair. Leave some space between the back of the chair and your back. Rock forward and back to find the sit bones. Feet flat on the floor, hip-distance apart. If you prefer, bring your knees together.

Bring your arms close to the side of your ribcage and put your palms together for namaste or clapping under your chest. Keep your shoulders rolled down away from the ears, and ensure your spine is erect, not hunched or bent. Inhale and exhale a few times, becoming aware of the posture. Exhale while tilting your neck towards your right shoulder as comfortably as possible. Pay conscious attention to how the right ear dips towards the right shoulder without raising the shoulder. As you take in breaths, feel the stretch along both sides of the neck and back. Afterward, return to the center with an inhale. Repeat on the other side, following your breath, still feeling into both sides of the neck and back when stretching. Engage with this movement five to six times on each side with ease and peace, according to your comfort level.

Wrist Joint Rotation

Manibandha Chakra

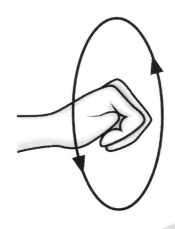

This strengthens the wrist's joints and increases movement.

Start off this practice by taking a comfortable seat. Sit up tall, shoulders relaxed. Bring your body and mind into a state of concentration on the joint movements. You can rotate both wrists together or one wrist at a time. Extend your arms forward parallel to the ground at shoulder level and lightly clench your hands into fists with thumbs tucked in. Direct the fists downward towards the floor. Gradually rotate them clockwise for five rotations and then counter-clockwise an additional five times. Make sure you keep your elbows held straight and hands shoulder-width apart from each other as you make broad circles with your wrists during the rotation process. Remember to move slowly and deliberately, staying aware of all sensations throughout this exercise.

Wrists Rotation Palms Up

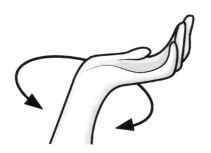

Open your fists up with your palms facing up.

Keep your elbows and arms straight. If your arms feel tired, then put them on the thighs. Take a couple of deep breaths and lift your arms in front of you in a previous position. Palms are facing up. Rotate your wrists for five rotations clockwise and switch to the other side.

Chair Upward Hand Stretch Pose

Urdhva Hastasana

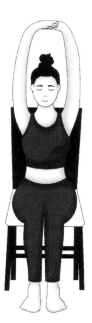

This pose helps the shoulders in flexion. When you lengthen the spine, the entire back muscles are stretched. Elbows, wrists, fingers, and neck are flexed to support the torso in this stretch.

Not only does it help with physical mobility, but it also promotes relaxation and breath awareness. The lungs, heart, and abdominal organs are activated by stretching the arms. As the armpits are extended, the lymph nodes are stimulated, facilitating the better circulation of blood and lymphatic fluid. As a result of stretching the side abdominal area, the digestive system can function better.

Sit up tall—ground through your sit bones on the chair, and ground your feet firmly on the floor. Connect to your breathing. Keep your back straight and long.

Check your feet; they should be parallel to the floor. Keep them a few inches away from each other. Check in with your breath and stay four to five breaths.

Once you're ready, bring your arms in front and lengthen. Interlock your fingers with palms facing outside and keep your arms stretched. Keep stretching and mindfully breathing for two to three breaths. Check that you're not lifting your shoulders. Imagine that you have loads of space between your shoulders and earlobes. Think that your neck is nice and tall.

When you're ready to move, inhale and raise your arms above your head. Keep fingers softly locked.

Hands are placed in line with the crown of the head. Exhale out fully.

Gently take the shoulders away from your ears. When they're touching your ears, the shoulders are not getting the full stretch they deserve.

Keep your gaze in front of you. Mindfully check if the hands are in line with the head and if the head is in line with the arms. Stretch as much as you can.

Exhale slowly and softly. Connect to your body. The stretch will become easy and comfortable with coordinated breath and body.

Remain in the stretch for about three to four or even four to six6 breaths, based on the body's comfort.

With every inhalation, go deeper upwards, and stretch more, but without causing tension to the neck and facial muscles. Smile.

To release, exhale and slowly lower the arms, coming back to the original position with the arms in front of you. Repeat this for the second round.

If this stretch feels too much, you can practice this by extending the arms up and bringing them down in reps of eight to ten, coordinating it with the breath. This will help energize your body and act as a warm-up for the shoulders, back, and abdomen.

Also, if this pose is not available for your body today, you can do it without interlocking the fingers.

Seated Palm Tree Pose Side Bend Flow Chair

Upavistha Parsva Bhanga Vinyasa

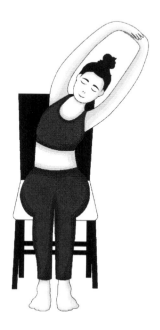

This asana strengthens, stretches, and lengthens the muscles between the ribs and hands (from shoulders to elbows to wrists and fingers), builds strength in arms and shoulders, and extends the abdominal muscles, hips, and thighs.

Sit up nice and tall. Feet are firmly on the ground, feel your body active, and don't tense up. Breathe in, and lift your heart to the sky.

Move at your own pace, follow your breath, and on the inhale, grow tall and reach both arms over your head by clasping fingers.

On the exhale, your hips remain on the chair and you bend from the waist to your right. Stay for one or two breaths.

Inhale, return to the center. On the exhale, bend from your waist to your left.

Chair Seated Side Stretch Pose

This is a quick way to relax the upper body and it helps to improve your balance. Stretches the muscles between the ribs, which helps to support them.

Inhale to lengthen the spine.

Reach the left arm up and over the ear, gently leaning across without moving too far.

Hold three breaths with your left hand up, right hand on the seat or left thigh. Exhale to slowly lower your arm before

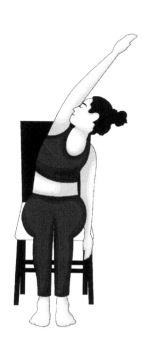

pausing to observe any bodily sensations. Listen to your body about how deep to go into the stretch.

Repeat with another side. Switch the arms and do it two to three times.

Eagle Arms

The muscles of the whole back are stretched, so it's a quick way to relieve shoulder and neck stiffness.

Sit comfortably on a chair, back straight, and feet firmly grounded on the floor. Take a few breaths here.

Cross the elbows, taking a right over left.

Interlock the arms. Bring your mind to the breath and stay for three breaths.

Release and repeat on the opposite side. Take and cross your left elbow over the right. Keep breathing for another three breaths. Release. Come back to the center.

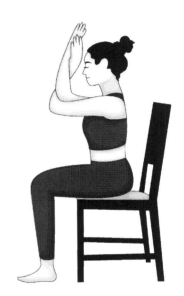

Seated Forward Fold Pose on Chair

Forward fold can quickly release tension in the upper body and help to open the lower back, shoulders, neck, and hips. It aids in removing the tightness and stiffness of the muscles. A quick way to awaken and open the upper body joints, nerves, and muscles. The forward fold will help stretch the lower back and the entire spine.

Note: If you have high blood pressure or difficulty breathing, you should not do this pose.

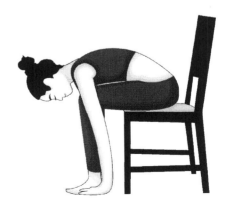

While seated in chair tadasana (Mountain Pose Chair), breathe in deep a few times to relax and extend the spine. Exhaling, bring your arms down towards your feet, with the torso resting on the thighs and chin close to the knees. Stretching the shoulders, place your palms flat on the floor and remain here for four breaths. As you exhale, push closer into the thighs and abdomen, stretching farther each time. To release, inhale, look up first, then raise your arms before coming back to sit in chair tadasana. Repeat this process as needed for a longer duration. Use a cushion for extra support if you need it under your chest and diaphragm.

Goddess Pose on Chair

Utkata Konasana

Sitting in this pose, you help to lengthen the spine by engaging the quadriceps, gluteus, hip flexors, inner thighs, and joints of the hips, knees, and feet when the arms are raised up.

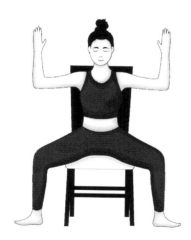

Sit nice and tall in the middle of the chair, leaving some space between your back and the backrest. Pressing through sits bones, open legs wide. Knees remain over ankles, and toes turn out slightly. Feel as if you're grounding through all four corners of your feet.

Feel the spine lengthen and keep an upright posture.

Extend arms and bend at the elbows with palms facing forward—cactus pose.

Squeeze your shoulder blades together slightly.

Lift chest up and outward. Feel the shoulder blades engage and the heart open.

To stay active in this pose, gently press through your heels and squeeze your shoulder blades.

Stay in the pose for a couple of cycles of breath, lower your arms and repeat another three times.

Chair Wide Legged Seated Twist

Usually, the twist helps open the heart, but sitting with legs comfortably wide also helps extend the hips.

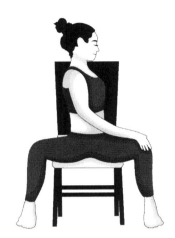

Remain seated in a goddess pose with arms lowered, with your knees wide open. Turn your toes slightly to face them forward, and stack your knees over your ankles. Tuck your tailbone in.

Both arms are resting on your thighs.

Breathe in, lengthening your spine, and twist towards the right.

The twist begins in your belly, ribs, and chest. Your head is last to turn.

Left hand goes onto your right knee and your right hand to the back of a chair. Breathe into the twist.

Stay here for three deep breaths.

Exhale to release and return to the center.

Repeat on the opposite side, each side twice.

Warrior Pose I Chair Variation

Upavistha Virabhadrasana I

The chair warrior is a great exercise to stretch your inner thighs, legs, glutes, and torso. It works your legs, buttocks, hips, and even arms.

Due to different body abilities, I have added three options to perform this pose.

Any option you choose to do, start by sitting up nice tall, with your spine straight, smile, and lift your heart up to the sky. Take a deep breath and exhale slowly.

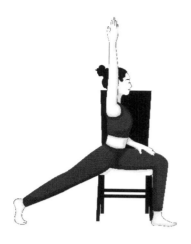

Move your left leg to the left. (Pic. 1)

Keep the left leg in over the side of the chair. Swing the right leg behind you. Pic. 1

Place the sole of the left foot on the floor roughly parallel to the chair's seat and straighten the right leg, supporting it with your toes. If this is not possible, slightly bend your right knee. Your torso is facing over the left leg. The left leg forms a nice 90-degree angle with knee stacked over the ankle. Your pelvis is engaged, the spine is straight, and the heart is lifted to the sky. Inhale as you raise your right arm to the ceiling. Left arm rest on your thigh.

Listen to your body. If this is too much, then do the pose in pic. 2.

Bring your right leg closer to your left leg. Breathe in and raise your arms over the head, palms facing each other.

If you can challenge your body more, you can try the pose in pic. 3.

Then when you move your right leg behind you, pay attention that you're coming onto the sole of your foot and both your arms are over your head with palms facing each other.

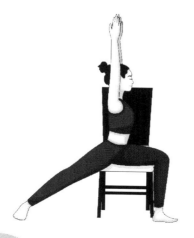

Breathe and listen. Find comfort in this position. When you breathe, pay attention so that your facial muscles are relaxed and there is no tension. Smile. Ensure that your shoulders are lowered, your neck is nice and tall, the heart is lifted, and the pelvis is engaged, holding you up.

Hold the pose for two to three breaths and come back to your seat. Repeat on the other side.

Chair Pigeon Pose

Chair Kapotasana

This pose helps open your hips, enhancing mobility and flexibility in the joint. In addition to stretching your hip flexors and lower back, pigeon pose alleviates mild lower back or hip pain by stretching these muscles regularly. A great way to ease the lower back stiffness, with the focus on stretching the hamstrings and the gluteus.

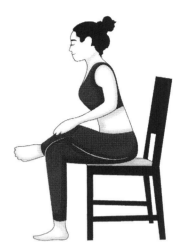

Sit nice and tall, with your back straight.

Now inhale and raise the right leg, holding it carefully with your hands and place it over the left thigh, sitting comfortably.

In this chair pigeon pose, the flexing of the hip joint and the knee play a role to keep them fit and flexible.

Once placed comfortably, sit straight if possible and take three breaths here, or as long as you need. If bringing the leg over and placing it on the other is difficult, then lift the right leg and try to hold it in your arms for a few seconds and then slowly release. Repeat with the opposite side.

Alternate-Nostril Breathing

Nadi Shodhana Pranayama

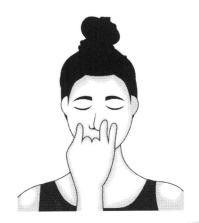

By activating your body's relaxation response, alternate-nostril breathing can help calm your body and mind.

Rest your left hand on your left thigh or in your lap or use it to support the elbow of your right arm. Close your right nostril with the thumb of that hand, inhale through the left, then close it off with your ring finger and pinky. Exhale through the right nostril for a short pause before repeating this cycle three to five times with both nostrils. When finished, return to regular breathing.

When you finish practice, sit with your eyes closed and your hands in your lap for a few minutes. Let your shoulders fall down and away from your ears. As you transition into the rest of your day, you will be able to absorb all the benefits of the poses you have done so far. Check how you feel. Breathe in through your nose and exhale through your mouth. Breathe in and feel the air traveling through your throat and to your belly. Open your mouth and exhale. Repeat for a couple of minutes.

Feel the sensations in your body right now. Warmth. Coolness. Tingling. Tightness. Pulsation. Relaxation. Hunger. Fullness. Observe the sensations in your body in this moment with patience and kindness. Explore both strong and subtle sensations with curiosity.

Your Chance to Help Someone Else

"Yoga is not to be performed;
It is to be lived.
Yoga doesn't care about what you have been;
It cares about the person you are becoming."

— *Aadil Palkhivala*

"I'm not flexible enough."

"I have back pain – there's no way I can do yoga."

"I'm too old to start practicing yoga now."

I can't tell you how many times I've heard these objections, not to mention a wealth of others. But as we saw in Chapter 3, there is a wealth of benefits to yoga… and the reality of chair yoga means that no one is excluded.

It's my goal to help as many people benefit from yoga as possible, and that starts with dispelling these myths and helping those who think they're too old, not flexible enough, or in too much pain, to realize that chair yoga is their solution.

You can help me spread the word – and just like chair yoga, it doesn't require much time or experience. All it takes is a few minutes and a few short sentences.

By leaving a review of this book on Amazon, you'll show other seniors just how beneficial yoga can be – and exactly where they can find all the guidance they need to make it accessible to them.

Simply by letting other readers know how this book has helped you and what they can expect to find inside, you'll signpost the route to a solution that could be life-changing for many people.

Thank you for your support. Yoga is for everyone, and all it takes to make it accessible – no matter what stage of life you're at – is the right guidance… and when you have that, it's amazing what benefits you can unlock.

Sequence Three
The Chair Yogi's Journey

Chair Mountain Pose Heel Raised

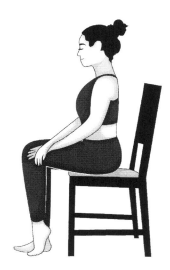

Sit nice and tall. Keep your shoulders relaxed. Your neck is nice and tall. Your arms can rest on your thighs. Take a few deep breaths. Check how you feel. Inhale and lift your one heel up. Take a couple of deep breaths. Lower on the exhale, repeat with the other foot.

Repeat five times for each foot and remember to coordinate it with a breath.

Wrist Rotations

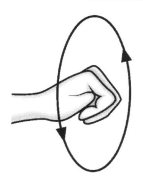

Lift your hands in front of you, parallel to the floor. You can lift both arms together and rotate both wrists at the same time or do one hand at a time.

Rotate your wrist five times clockwise and counterclockwise. Repeat five times for each wrist.

Don't forget to breathe; observe your body, listen to it.

Wrist Exercise Side to Side Close Up

After rotating your wrists, point fingers up straight, move your wrist to the left and then to the right.

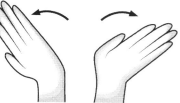

Repeat for both hands.

Breathe in and notice if your shoulders remain in the same position or try to move, too. Only the wrist should be moving.

Palms Stretch

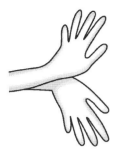

Keep sitting comfortably on the chair. Breathe. Press your palms away—imagine that you're pushing against the wall. Exhale, keep your hand straight and point your fingers to the floor.

Repeat five to ten times for each hand.

Bear Hug Stretch Pose Close Up

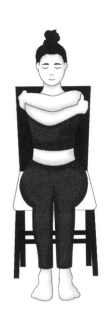

The hug will help to stretch your upper back and shoulders.

On the inhale, hug yourself.

Hold on to your shoulders as you open up your upper back while keeping your spine and back straight. Take a couple of deep breaths.

Chair Neck Stretch

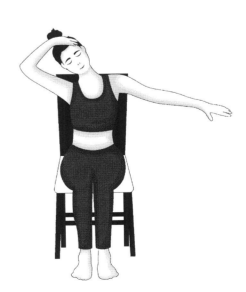

You will improve flexibility, mobility, and range of motion by practicing neck stretches. It also helps to reduce tension and stiffness in the neck.

Sit comfortably in the middle of the chair. Leave some space between the chair and your back.

Knees are stacked over your ankles, forming 90 degrees between your knees and hip.

Breathe in, and on your breath out, tilt your head towards your right shoulder, and place your right hand gently on the left ear. Extend your left arm. Stay and take a couple of deep breaths. You can breathe out with a slightly opened mouth.

Breathe in your nose and return to the center with arms lying on your knees or thighs.

On the exchange, tilt your head towards your left shoulder and place your left hand gently on the right ear. Extend your right arm. Stay there and take a couple of deep breaths.

Repeat another two times.

Eagle Pose Chair

Garudasana

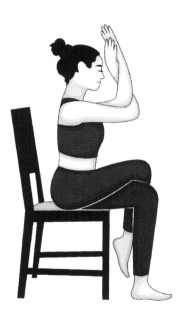

This pose is good to get whole back muscles stretched, so it's a quick way to relieve shoulder and neck stiffness. As the legs are crossed, it also helps to loosen up your knees.

Sit up tall with your back straight.

Cross the left leg over the right knee. If you can't cross high in your legs, then cross low in your legs (shins or ankles). If you can, then tuck the left toes around your right calf. Don't force yourself into the position.

Bring your arms in front of you.

Take your left elbow and hook it underneath the right elbow.

Sit and hold for a couple of deep breaths. Feel the stretch.

Shoulder Socket Rotation

Skandha Chakra

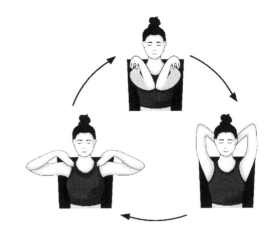

With the elbows bent, shoulder rolls strengthen the rotator cuff muscles, strengthening the shoulder joint. In addition to preventing injuries, this provides a solid foundation for poses requiring shoulder strength. Shoulder rolls with bent elbows can effectively aid in combating diseases and ailments caused by aging, such as osteoporosis and rheumatoid arthritis.

Note: If you had an injury or surgery in a shoulder area, don't practice this without consulting your physician.

Sit up tall with your back straight. Bring the fingertips to rest on the shoulders.

On the inhale, begin to move the bent elbows from the center, moving upwards.

Move them in a circular movement from the center about six times.

Repeat the opposite direction another six times.

Watch your breath, and work on coordinating the action with your breath at your own pace.

Elbow Bending Close Up

Kehuni Nama Close

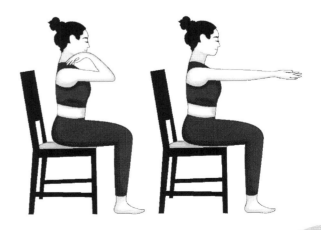

This exercise is a warm-up to your arms and will help to boost energy in the body. Also, it will help to build flexibility in your elbows.

Sit up tall with your back straight.

Both feet are touching the ground. Lift your heart to the sky and tuck your pelvis in.

Both knees are together, and your arms are stretched in front of you. Palms are facing up.

On the inhale, bend the elbows and bring the fingers to your shoulders.

Exhale—repeat this motion, moving the fingers from the front to the shoulder and then extending the arms back in front of you.

Inhale and exhale. Repeat this about ten times with each arm.

Arms Swing Pose Flow Close Up

Hasta Swing Vinyasa

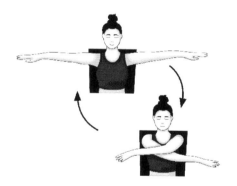

Exercises like arm swings warm up and stretch the shoulders, arms, chest, and upper back, preparing the muscles, tendons, and joints for other poses.

Raise your arms sideways, parallel to the floor.

Allow your arms to swing forward, hands crossing over each other.

Swing arms back, then forward again, alternating which hand swings over the top of the other.

This movement may not be in time with your breath, and that is okay.

Goddess Pose Chair Side Stretch

As the nature of the pose, the Goddess Pose Chair Side Stretch helps to open the shoulders, upper back, chest, and neck when the arms are stretched to the opposite way, and open the hips and whole pelvis. In addition to stretching the psoas and strengthening the knees and ankles on the chair, this pose strengthens the knees and ankles by keeping the legs active and wide without putting too much stress on them.

Sit up tall, closer to the edge of the chair.

Open the legs wide, firm on the ground, with feet pointing out.

Rest the right elbow on the right thigh, the palm facing up.

On inhale, sweep the left arm up, look up if you can, and gaze at the hand.

Breathe deeply here for three breaths. Repeat on the other side.

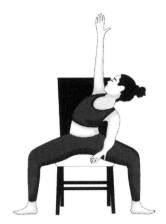

Revolved Chair Pose on Chair

Parivrtta Utkatasana

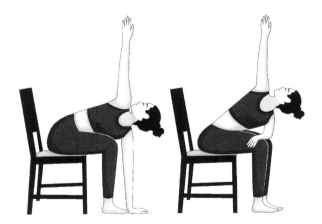

Revolved Chair Pose Chair Variation

Elbow Thighs

Besides stretching and opening the chest, shoulders, and upper back, the revolved chair pose strengthens the glutes, thighs, ankles, calves, and lower back. This pose increases balance and focus and improves joint mobility.

Start in a mountain pose with your spine straight and roll back the shoulders. Think of a tall neck; the heart is lifted towards the sky. Deep breaths. Inhale and extend the spine, exhale, and bend forward, reaching for the ground with the left arm. Rest your palm on the floor; if this is not possible, lean onto your fingers. Don't put all your weight onto them. The core is active and supports you too. Inhale as you raise the right arm up and exhale looking up at the extended limb. Stay here for two to three deep breaths and repeat on another side.

If this is not possible and the body feels uncomfortable, try another variation, with your left elbow resting on the top of the knee—revolved chair pose chair variation elbow thighs. Do exactly the same, just instead of placing your arm on the floor, bend your elbow and place it on the knees. Check with your body—spine is long, neck is straight and you're looking up at the top of your fingers.

Bharadvaja's Twist

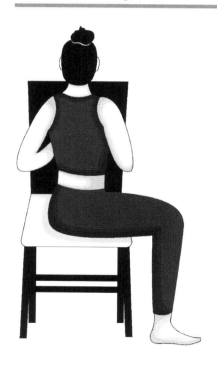

You should sit sideways on the edge of a chair, with your left side close to the chair's back. Your feet should be parallel and your knees directly above your ankles.

Imagine that you have a block between your knees, or you can use an actual yoga one and squeeze it. You should feel a pressure transfer up your inner thighs and firm your core.

Make space in your spine by lengthening your back. Press the sitting bones into the chair to sit upright, with the crown of your head directly over the spinal column. Exhale and let go of your shoulder blades as you lift your head up to the ceiling. On an inhale, lift up the sides of your navel area and then exhale to draw it towards your spine.

Turn towards the left and place hands on the back of the chair while rotating ribcage. Notice if either shoulder haa tensed, then move lower left shoulder blade towards spine and right one away from it. Rotate as far as possible, turn head to right side and extend left collarbone towards left shoulder, followed by another turn of head over left shoulder. Repeat process on the right side, both times deeper than first twist for a more enjoyable experience.

Seated Low Lunge Pose

Upavistha Anjaneyasana

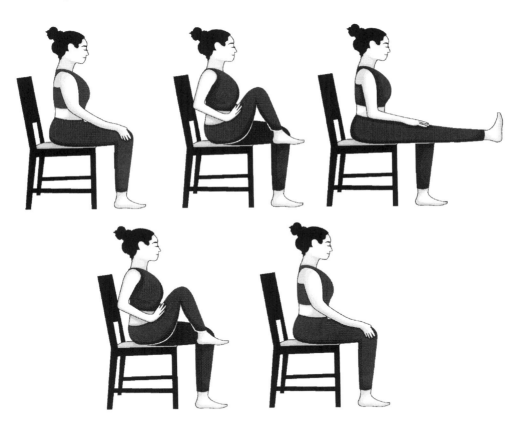

This easy flow will help stretch your feet, ankles, hips, and knees, and strengthen your pelvic floor.

Sitting tall with both feet on the floor, sit bones grounded on the chair.

Inhale and bend your right knee towards your chest.

Exhale and extend your leg out. Toes up toward the ceiling. Inhale, and bring it back by bending your right knee towards your chest. Exhale and place your foot on the floor.

Repeat on the other side, five total for each leg.

If you need to bend your knee towards your chest, you can grab under the knee and support your move.

Chair Pigeon Pose Variation Forward Bend

Chair Kapotasana Variation Uttanasana Namaste

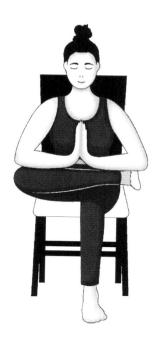

This is an excellent pose to flex tight hamstrings, hip flexors, glutes, and lower back or even the psoas muscles. This pose works to enhance the mobility of your knees, hips, pelvic girdle, and ankles by folding the leg and bending forward.

Begin the pose by comfortably sitting in chair tadasana (chair mountain pose) with feet touching the ground, back straight with a long spine, and soft breathing.

On the inhale, bring the right ankle to rest on the left thigh with your hands, keeping the knee in line with your ankle as much as possible. The left leg is grounded with the flat foot in chair pigeon pose. Use both hands to adjust the position of the ankle on the other knee.

Breathe and lengthen the spine. Feel the hip flexors contracting and the joint of the hips, knee, and ankle being active. Engage the pelvic floor muscles and remain here for about four to five breaths, consciously pushing the right knee down (but without using the hands).

Inhale and bring the hands in front of your chest, palms facing each other. Keep forearms parallel to the ground.

As you exhale, go for a forward bend from the hips to intensify the stretch. Engage the pelvic muscles. Try bringing the chest closer to the thighs. Breathe, and observe how your body feels—moving forward when exhaling.

Find the spot until you can't go farther, and once comfortable, hold for about three to four breaths. If you can, on the exhale, go deeper into the forward bend. If you cannot, then stay where you are. Remember to keep your spine long, shoulder relaxed, and away from your ears.

To release, inhale, lift your head and come up to straight back, exhale, release the hands, and with the support of hands, release the right leg and relax.

Now inhale, and bring the left ankle to rest on the right thigh, keeping the knee in line with your ankle as much as possible. The right leg is grounded with the foot flat. And repeat the same steps.

Warrior Pose II Chair

Virabhadrasana Ii Chair

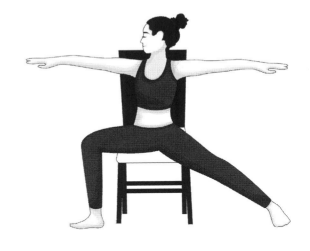

This strengthens and stretches your legs, ankles and feet. Stretches your hips, groin and shoulders. Develops stamina and concentration, balance and stability.

Begin the pose by comfortably sitting in chair tadasana (chair mountain pose) with feet touching the ground, back straight with a long spine, and soft breathing.

Sit on the edge of the chair. Stay here for two to three breaths.

Inhale, and separate the feet. Starting on the left first, open the left leg like goddess pose, but the left leg only. The knee aligns with the ankle and hip, forming a 90-degree angle. The foot is flat and relaxed, with the toes pointing to the left. Exhale and extend the right leg behind to make it straight in the knee. Here, the right foot is flat, and the toes point to the front.

With the hands resting on the knees, make your back straight and erect. Sit nice and tall. Once the body is comfortable, inhale and extend your arms at shoulder level to a nice T.

Ensure the palms are face down and elbows are not bent.

Finally, turn your head and gaze at your left fingers. Ensure the spine is erect and the chest and shoulders are open.

While here, check the alignment of the legs—the front knee doesn't drop to the side. Stay balanced in the pose. Breathe slowly, deeply, and softly.

To release the pose:

Turn your head back to the center on the exhale.

Lower your hands and realign your legs to chair tadasana.

Stay here for a while.

Following the previous steps, counter the stretch on the other side (right).

Humble Warrior Pose Chair

Baddha Virabhadrasana Chair

Humble warrior has the same benefits as warrior II. It's also a great way to keep the mind tranquil and balance unwanted emotions. This is powerful grounding posture also encourages energy flow and opens up the hips for a forward bend. It boosts blood circulation around the pelvic area.

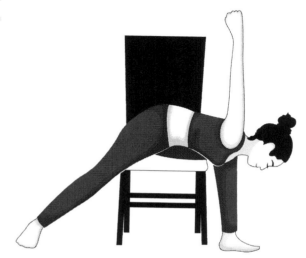

Note: This pose should be avoided if you had an injury or a surgery to shoulders, wrists, neck, hips, knees, lower back, ankles, feet or pelvis.

Sit nice and tall. Remember to breathe deeply.

Turn your body to the left with your left leg bent over the seat of the chair. Place the left leg in L shape. The right leg is stretched out behind you to the right side of the chair, with the foot flat and relaxed, and the toes point to the front. Extend the spine upward, pulling the belly in and lifting the pelvic floor. Gently interlace your fingers behind your back. Inhale and expand your chest and as you exhale, firmly press all four corners of the feet towards the ground. Take another deep breath, pull the arms behind you, and turn the chest and shoulders towards the left side, facing the left foot. As you exhale, come in a forward bend from the hips, gently move towards the left side, keep the chest and shoulders in a twist towards the left, extend the arms behind you upwards and bring the head towards the left foot.

Do not droop the neck and head. Think about your neck and head as an extension of your spine.

To release, inhale, look up first, and lift the neck and chest. Inhale, lift the entire torso and come back to the center. With the feet still firmly grounded, release the lock of the hands.

If this feels too challenging to your body at this time, move on to another humble warrior variation.

Humble Warrior Pose Chair Variation

Baddha Virabhadrasana Chair

Keep the exact alignment of your legs as in the previous pose.

Turn your body to the left with your left leg bent over the seat. Place the left leg in L shape. The right leg is stretched out behind you to the right side of the chair, with the foot flat and relaxed and the toes pointing front. Extend the spine upward,

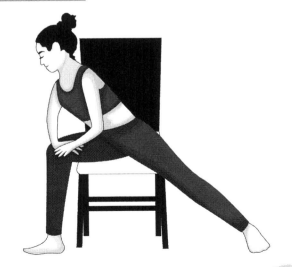

pulling the belly in and lifting the pelvic floor. Place your palms on your left knee. Take two to three breaths and repeat on another side.

Firefly Pose

Tittibhasana

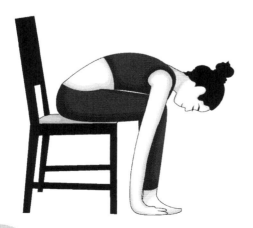

Sit up tall, closer to the edge of the chair.

Open the legs wide, firm on the ground, with feet pointing out.

On the front of the chair seat, bring your hands to rest.

Check your spine—lengthen it, engage your abs, and press your hands firmly into the chair seat as if you were going to lift your body off the chair.

Activate your quads to straighten both legs and lift your feet off the floor. Take a few breaths if you can, and lower the legs down.

If you cannot lift both legs simultaneously, try to raise only one and repeat two to three times for each leg.

Find what is comfortable for you.

Seated Forward Fold Pose on Chair

Forward fold can quickly release tension in the upper body and help to open the lower back, shoulders, neck, and hips. It aids in removing the tightness and stiffness of the muscles. A quick way to awaken and open the upper body joints, nerves, and muscles. The forward fold will help stretch the lower back and the entire spine.

Note: If you have high blood pressure or difficulty breathing, you should not do this pose.

While seated in chair tadasana (mountain pose chair), breathe in deep for a few times to relax and extend the spine. Exhaling, bring your arms down towards your feet, with the torso resting on the thighs and chin close to the knees. Stretching the shoulders, place your palms flat on the floor and remain here for four breaths. As you exhale, push closer into the thighs and abdomen, stretching farther each time. To release, inhale, look up first, then raise your arms before coming back to sit in chair tadasana. Repeat this process as needed for a longer duration. Use a cushion for extra support under your chest and diaphragm if you need help.

You can also try the variation of forward fold. (Pic 1 and Pic 2) The idea is to give you the option to be able to adjust to your body's needs at the present time.

If you cannot go all the way down and touch the floor, or you feel tension in your back, try half of forward fold with your arms on your knees or crossed.

The aim is to release the tension and to open the lower back. Breathe, listen to your body and choose the position that you feel comfortable in.

Seated Half Forward Fold Pose Chair (Pic 1) or

Seated Forward Fold Pose Chair Variation Arms Crossed (Pic 2)

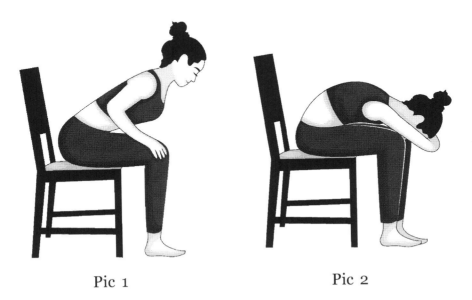

Pic 1

Pic 2

Seated Corpse Pose

Savasana

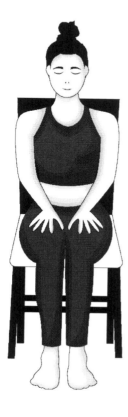

Sit up straight. You can rest your back on the chair. Sit the way you feel comfortable.

Observe where your hands are. Support your hands in your lap or place them gently, palm down, on your knees.

Find a comfortable position and keep your eyes open with a soft gaze or closed. Take long, slow, deep breaths through your nose, inhaling fully and exhaling fully. Allow your breath to find its natural rhythm of in-breath and out-breath movement. Tune in to the sensations that come with each breath. Notice what the air is like when entering your nose. Is it cool? Is it warm when you exhale? Let go of any external noises around you and focus on nothing but your breathing. If distracted by thought patterns, observe them without judgment or expectation to change them; notice them float away like leaves down a stream before bringing yourself back to focusing on the breath. Pay attention to the rise of your stomach on the inhale and the relaxation on the exhale. Acknowledge any pain, discomfort, or feelings that arise during this practice without judgment or clinging onto them—rather, refocus back to your breathing when necessary. As this practice ends, slowly expand your awareness to take in the entire body, finally returning fully alert to your environment. Establish an intention to use this practice daily to cultivate strong focus and attentiveness.

Sequence Four
The Dance of Yoga

Seated Five-Pointed Star Pose Chair

Utthita Tadasana Chair

Let's take a couple of deep breaths and dive into your practice. Boost your energy with the five-pointed star pose chair.

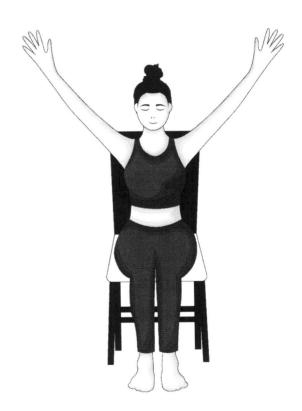

Sit in your chair. Move forward, so your feet are flat on the floor, your back is straight, and your spine is elongated. Tuck your chin in slightly. Pull shoulders away from the ears, shoulder blades going down the back. The crown of the head should be reaching towards the ceiling.

On an inhale, lift your arms in a Y. Spreads your fingers.

On exhale, lower back down and make a light fist of them. On the inhale, lift your arms and spread your fingers.

Repeat three to five times.

Or, you can lift your arms in a Y shape, keep them there for a few breaths, and lower them down. Listen to your body and do what feels good.

Chair Mountain Pose Sweeping Arms Flow

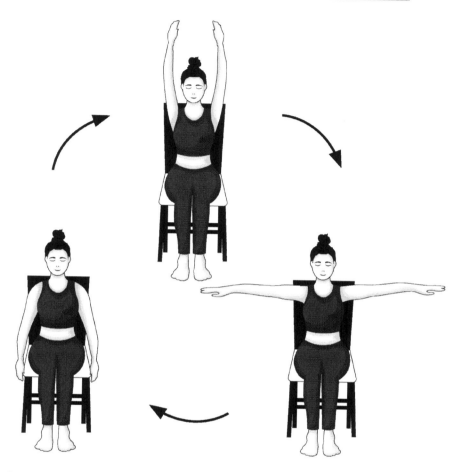

This will help you to warm up your shoulders.

Sit in a mountain pose. Inhale reaching the arms up, palms facing each other above your head. Exhale and slowly release them down, palms facing down. Inhale reaching the arms up; exhale palms face down. Repeat the sequence for another two or three times.

Arms to Side Rotations Chair

Parsva Hasta Paryayakrama Chair

This movement also belongs to the warm-up, which will help to prepare your arms and wrists.

On your inhale, bring your arms up and position them to your sides, parallel to the floor.

Exhale and slowly rotate your arms in large circles for a few rotations.

Breathe. Bring your arms back to your legs.

Inhale and bring your arms back up, exhale, and rotate in the opposite direction.

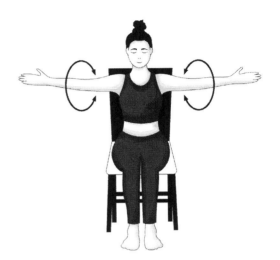

Goddess Pose on Chair Arms Flow

Utkata Konasana on Chair Hasta

This flow will assist with more significant expansion, helping to improve your breathing. This gentle flow practice will assist in easing your back pain, also reducing stiffness in your shoulders and neck.

Sit in your chair. Move forward, so your feet are flat on the floor, your back is straight, and your spine is elongated. Tuck your chin in slightly. Pull shoulders away from the ears, shoulder blades going down the back. The crown of the head should be reaching towards the ceiling.

Inhale to rotate the hips outwards, bringing the feet to 120 degrees, with toes pointing sideways and knees bent.

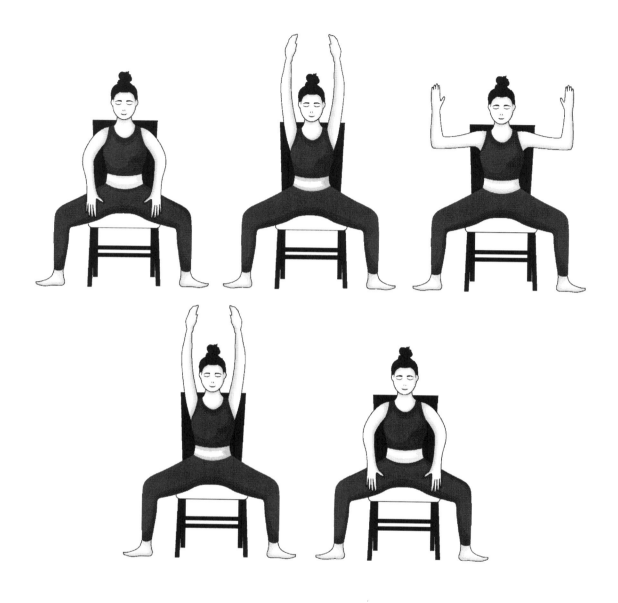

Gently push out the inner thighs as you plant both feet firmly on the floor. Raise your arms overhead—palms facing each other—keeping shoulders away from ears. Exhale while bending elbows so forearms are perpendicular and palms are facing forward (cactus arms). Hold for thirty seconds before inhaling to extend arms up again with palms together. Lower arms back down at shoulder level in an exhale and place hands on inner thighs before inhaling again to raise them. Complete four to six repetitions of this flow, coordinating breathing as needed, then release and relax.

Once you will complete it, remain in the goddess pose for your next pose.

Goddess Pose Chair Hands Behind Head Side Bend

Parsva Utkata Konasana Chair Hasta Sirsa

The back is long and the shoulders are away from the ears and you're sitting in the goddess pose, with knees and hips opened wide.

On the inhale, lift your arms and put them behind your head. Press away from the ground. Keep your elbows opened. Inhale and slightly pull your shoulder blades back.

On the exhale from the torso, bend to the right. You can stay in this position for one or two breaths or come back to the middle on your inhale. And repeat. On the exhale, repeat it on another side. Do a few cycles on each side.

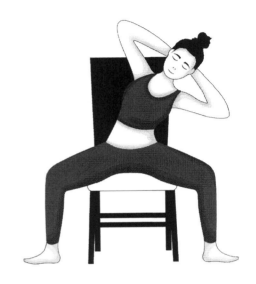

Revolved Goddess Pose

Sit up nice and tall. Pull shoulders away from the ears, shoulder blades going down the back. The crown of the head should be reaching towards the ceiling. Move back and forward to find and feel your sit bones. Breathe in and open the legs wide, like for a goddess pose. Check that your knees align with the hips and ankles, forming a 90-degree angle. Place your hand on the thighs. Bring your heels slightly in and turn the toes slightly out. Roll the shoulders back.

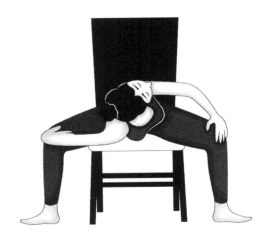

Inhale, place your hands on the knees, and slowly bend forward on the exhale, with your back parallel to the ground.

Twist to the left first, inhale, and draw the navel into the spine. While exhaling, twist the torso to the left. Take the left shoulder back and the right forward.

Stay here for up to six breaths or as long as comfortable, twisting your neck to fix your gaze over the shoulder.

To release, inhale, release the twist and forward bend, and come back to the center. Take a few breaths and as you're ready, exhale and, this time, twist and turn to another side. Bring the right shoulder back and the left forward.

Chair Mountain Pose Stand Up Flow

Chair Tadasana Samasthiti Vinyasa

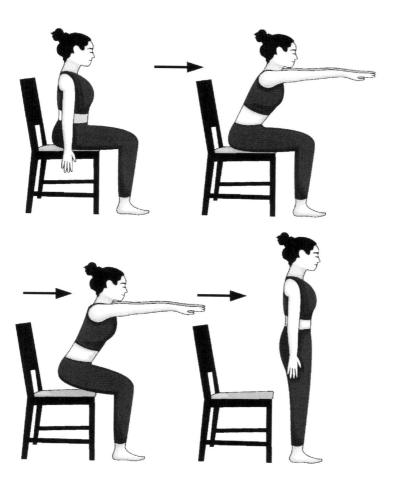

This practice is good as it strengthens the knees, hamstrings, lower back, and hips. Without putting too much pressure on the base of the spine and with the help of soft breathing, this pose can aid in easing back pains.

Start in a tadasana.

The spine is nice and tall, shoulders rolled back. Reach your arms forward to help you lift your hips off the chair. Hold this position for a couple of breaths; if not, stand up. Feel the ground under your feet. Sit back down with your arms next to you. Repeat three more times.

Chair Pose Hovering Above Chair

Utkatasana Hovering Above Chair

Sit up nice and tall. Pull shoulders away from the ears, shoulder blades going down the back. The crown of the head should be reaching towards the ceiling. Move back and forward to find and feel your sit bones.

Raise your arms above the head and exhale.

On the inhale, stand up on your feet in chair pose, hovering above the chair. Inhale through your nose and breathe out loudly through your mouth.

On the exhale, sit back on the chair. Keep your arms above your head.

Inhale and come back to chair pose again.

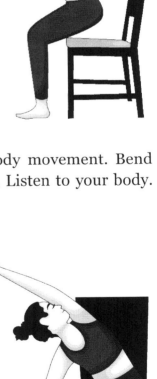

Repeat this six times. Try to coordinate your breath with body movement. Bend the knees and don't push or stretch the arms beyond comfort. Listen to your body.

Gate Pose on Chair

Parighasana on Chair

Shift your hips towards the right side of your chair, closer to the edge. Make sure that you're still sitting stable on the chair.

On the inhale, extend your right leg, nice and long, and press the foot to the floor with your toes pointing forward. Keep the left knee firmly over the ankle.

Take a few breaths here as you extend the spine upwards. Inhale, raise the left arm above your head, stretching towards the right side. Exhale, stretch entirely, and look up.

Your right arm can rest on your right thigh, knee, or shin, whichever feels good. Remain in this posture for six breaths or as long as you can. On the inhale, come back to the center. Repeat on the opposite side. Repeat one more time, twice on each side in total. If your body feels uncomfortable, go back to the center and try again or move to another pose.

Seated Revolved Arms Extended Eagle Legs Pose

Parivrtta Upavistha Hasta

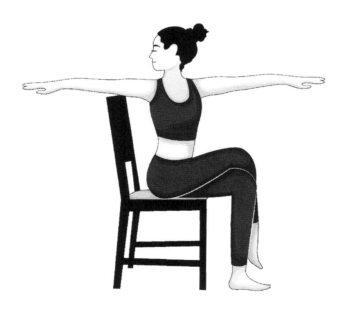

This pose strengthens your core, thighs, legs, and ankles, and it stretches your shoulders, upper back, and thighs.

Sit up nice and tall. Pull the shoulders away from the ears, and roll the shoulder blades back. The crown of the head should reach toward the ceiling. Move back and forward to find and feel your sit bones. Put your right leg over your left leg.

On the inhale, lift your heart to the sky. Extend your arms to a T, and on the exhale, twist your torso to the right, the head looking over your right shoulder, arms being straight, at the shoulder level, parallel to the floor. Stay in the pose for three breaths. On the exhale, release. Repeat on the other side.

Seated External Hip Rotation Pose Cactus Arms Chair

Upavishta External Hip Rotation Cactus Arms Chair

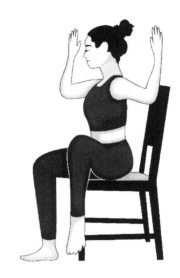

Draw the crown of your head towards the sky and lengthen your spine. Place your hands gently on your knees. Sit up nice and tall. Shoulders are relaxed; the spine is straight. Feel like you're grounding through the hips and feet.

Cactus arms, elbows in line with shoulders, wrists stacked over elbows. Spread the fingers and point them up. Breathe in and bring your arms to the side with your elbows bent as pictured.

Inhale and check that your core is active, the neck is long, and the shoulder blades are down the back.

On the inhale, bring the right leg out towards the right side, and on the exhale, bring it back to the center. Repeat eight to ten times with one leg.

If your arms are tired, release your cactus arms and take a few breaths in mountain pose. Repeat on the other side.

Seated Crescent Low Lunge Pose Variation Arms Sway Chair

Upavistha Anjaneyasana
Variation Hasta Sway Chair

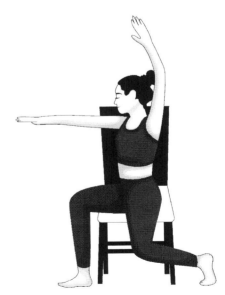

Sit nice and tall. Abdominals are engaged. Breathe in and imagine that you're lifting your heart up. Tuck your chin slightly in. Check if your upper body makes a nice angle with your hips, the same as the hips make a nice angle to your knees.

Sit towards the edge of the seat and turn both knees to the left until the left thigh is parallel with the front edge of the seat. The left knee is facing to the left; the left ankle is under the left knee. Reach with the left hand for the back of the chair. Sitting tall, torso extended, crown to the sky, begin to reach the right foot back until the right knee is under the right hip (entire right leg off the chair, right sit bone on the edge of the seat).

Hug the right inner thigh toward the chair. Push the back toes into the earth, and keep the front foot firmly on the ground. Engage the glutes and keep the pelvis level, trying not to lean to one side. Imagine that all the weight is equally distributed in your body.

Inhale, lengthen the torso, and pull shoulders away from ears, then exhale and move the right arm forward and up beside the right ear, palm facing inward. Extend the torso, eyes straight ahead, chin in line with the heart center. Stay in this position for three breaths. On the exhale, slowly release and repeat on the other side.

You can repeat it again if you wish.

Chair Hand to Big Toe Pose

Chair Padangusthasana

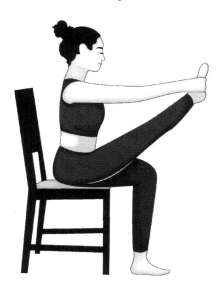

This pose helps to stretch and strengthen hamstrings, calves, glutes, and quadriceps, as well as activate the core abdominal muscles, which helps to improve balance.

Sit nice and tall. Feel your abdominals engaged, and check that your spine is straight and your shoulders relaxed. On the inhale, bend your right knee and take your right foot into your hands, or hold on to your ankle or shin, and on the exhale, try to stretch your right foot and maintain your straight back. Don't lock your knee; slightly bend it. Don't force yourself into the pose. Stretch your foot as much as you can today. Remain in the pose for two to three breaths, gently bend your right knee on the exhale and put your foot down. Repeat on the other side. Repeat the cycle twice for each leg.

Boat Pose Variation on Chair

Navasana Variation on Chair

The pose will help to develop stronger abdominal muscles which will aid you in a better posture, better digestion, reduce back pain and better sleep.

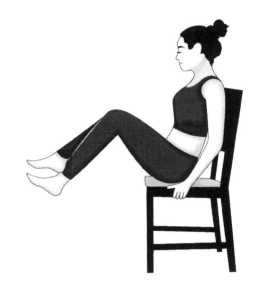

Draw the crown of your head towards the sky and lengthen your spine. Place your hands gently on your knees. Sit up nice and tall. Shoulders are relaxed; the spine is straight. Feel like you're grounding through the hips and feet.

On the inhale, grab the chair's sides with your hands. The hands are placed right behind the buttocks. The four fingers curl underneath the chair, and the thumb rests on top of the chair, near the buttocks. While doing this, the weight is on the outer edges of the palms. Ensure the chest is broad and the shoulders are dropped behind, rolling them away from the ears. The upper body is neutral—the shoulder blades don't move away from or toward each other.

On the exhale, lift the feet off the mat, keeping the knees bent. Keep the legs together by squeezing the inner thighs and crossing the ankles if possible. The ankles are in line with the seat of the chair.

Inhale and lengthen the spine as you draw the abdomen to bear the legs' weight. The body will lean back naturally, which should help keep the chest open as you engage your navel. The hands on the chair should help with balancing and reduce the pressure on the lower back.

Ensure that the lower back does not curl up. This can be done by being conscious of the pelvic floor and core. As you engage the core, take awareness of the pelvic floor. To maintain a straight spine, keep trying to ground yourself on the chair with the sit bones. Breathe. Even as you lean back and lift the legs, keep trying to send the sit bones to the chair. This will help in maintaining a straight back. Remain here for three to four breaths.

To release the pose, uncross the ankles and send your feet down one after another. If you feel the tension in your neck, gently do a few neck rolls.

If you feel the tension in your back, do the cat and cow pose from previous sequences.

If you cannot lift both legs simultaneously, do everything the same, but instead of lifting both legs, lift one leg with the opposite leg remaining on the floor. Stay for three to four breaths and switch the legs.

Standing Table Top Pose with Knee to Nose

Tada Bharmanasana Knee To Nose Vinyasa Chair

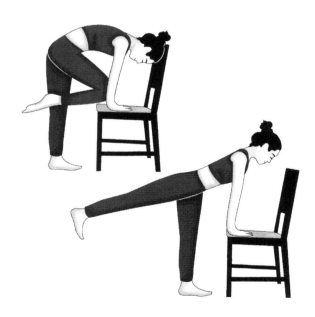

This pose will help you to build strength and stability in your legs and hips. Extending the leg back is a great way to open the lower back muscles.

Stand up tall and straight, facing the seat of the chair.

Take a couple of deep breaths.

On the inhale, place your hands on the chair. Exhale and extend the arms; think that your neck is the expression of your spine.

Exhale and lengthen through your spine and head.

Inhale and take the right leg behind you and extend the foot as much as you can. Bring the right knee to your nose on the exhale as you bend it.

On the inhale, take the leg back by extending it, exhale, and bring it back to your nose. Repeat this flow six times on one side.

Return to a standing mountain pose and repeat on the other side.

Seated Windshield Wiper Pose Chair

This movement will help you to loosen up your hips and knees.

Sit up straight and tall. Keep your legs wide apart. Take a few breaths to the windshield wiper, your knees in and out, moving side to side with your breath at your own pace, releasing the tension.

Come back to center.

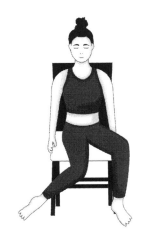

Chair Roll Down Pose

Sit up straight and tall. Drop your chin to your chest. Let your back relax into a rounded position. Move your hands down the front of your shins but only as far as is comfortable. Take a deep breath in a fold position and slowly return. Initiate the movement from your lower, middle, and upper back, and lift your head. Listen to your body and repeat the roll down slowly. Once you're in a forward fold, stay here for a few breaths and then slowly and gently roll back to the center.

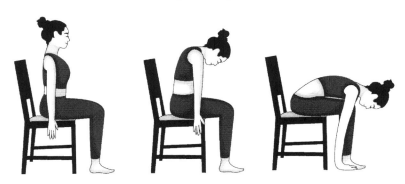

Cool Down

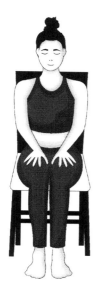

Sit nice and tall. You can rest your back on the backrest but aim to keep it straight.

Keep your arms together on your thighs or knees. Close your eyes or soften your gaze.

Feel supported by the chair beneath you.

Is there anything that you could adjust? How does your body feel?

Touch your arm and wish yourself well. Say in your mind or out loud that you love yourself as you are and you're enough.

Wiggle your toes and feel the ground supporting your feet.

Let your thoughts float in the air, thank them for turning up and let them pass. Notice if there is any tension in the back or shoulders. If you can feel any, then take a deep breath and soften. Lift your shoulders up and release. Bring your attention back to the room. Listen to the sounds around you, and when you're ready, open your eyes. Don't rush off the chair. Stand up when you're ready.

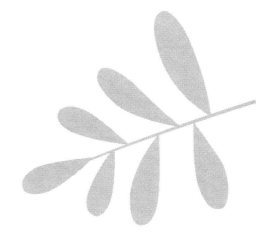

Chapter 8

Chapter 8 has back pain, achy joints, headaches, migraines, and neck tension relief sequences.

You can perform them as a stand-alone or combine them with others.

For example, you can choose one breathing exercise from chapter 5, one warm-up sequence from chapter 6, and, depending on your pain, one from chapter 8. You will be familiar with some poses as you have performed them before; some will be new.

You don't have to feel pain in your body to open chapter 8 and practice.

These sequences can be practiced as prevention too.

They've been created to stretch and loosen up the muscles, which cause pain due to their stiffness.

Back Pain Relief Sequence

Rotating the neck will help to release the tension built around the neck and the shoulders. Stiffness around the neck and shoulders could cause headaches that could lead to a lack of sleep.

Come back to chair tadasana (mountain pose).

Center and relax for a few breaths.

If there is discomfort in the head due to movement of the neck, take deep breaths through both nostrils.

Inhale and lengthen through your spine. Ground down through the sit bones and imagine how the crown of your head rises towards the ceiling.

Tuck your chin in slightly.

Inhale and move your head to the right and exhale.

On the inhale, come back to the center, exhale, and pause before switching sides.

Repeat on another side: inhale, move your head to the left, relax, and exhale. Then inhale and return to the center.

Repeat two to four times for each side.

Chair Cat-Cow Pose

Chair Marjaryasana Bitilasana

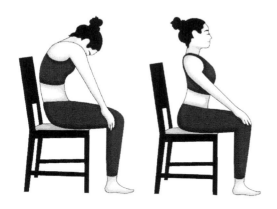

Chair cat-cow pose is an effective way to tackle back pain and neck and shoulder stiffness. This therapeutic practice boosts flexibility as it stretches and massages the abdominal cavity, helping to improve digestion. Additionally, it increases the oxygenated blood supply in the spine, allowing a smoother and less painful movement of the back and neck muscles. Those with rheumatoid arthritis or osteoarthritis can benefit from this pose as the regular practice may help prevent these conditions from developing and reduce their symptoms at early stages.

Note: If you have a neck injury, shoulders, spine, or hip injury, or have had recent abdominal surgery, you should avoid practicing the cat-cow pose and check with your doctor first.

Also, please **do not round** your spine if you have osteopenia or osteoporosis. On your exhale—return to a **neutral spine** instead of rounding. Sit in a mountain pose. Relax and connect to your breath. Sit up tall. Feel the crown of your head rising towards the ceiling. Connect to your breath and take a couple of deep breaths. Rest your feet on the floor and keep your knees aligned with your hips.

Put your arms on your knees.

On the inhale, expand your chest. Let your head and chin go slightly back.

On the exhale, round your spine by curling the chest in.

Check if your shoulders are relaxed. Feel the space between your shoulders and earlobes. Keep breathing.

Practice coordinating your breath with movement. Don't rush. Smile, inhale, and repeat the movement three to five times.

Eagle Arms

Muscles of the whole back are stretched, so it's a quick way to relieve shoulder and neck stiffness.

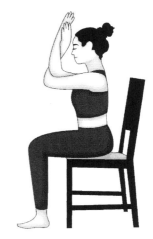

Sit comfortably on a chair, back straight and feet firmly grounded on the floor. Take a few breaths here.

Cross the elbows, taking a right over left.

Interlock the arms. Bring your mind to the breath and stay for three breaths.

Release and repeat on the opposite side. Take and cross your left elbow over the right. Keep breathing for another three breaths. Release. Come back to the center.

Eagle Pose Chair

Garudasana

This pose is good to get all the back muscles stretched, so it's a quick way to relieve shoulder and neck stiffness. As the legs are crossed, it also helps to loosen up your knees.

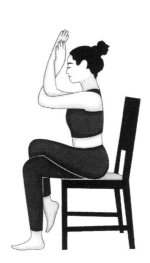

Sit up tall with your back straight.

Cross the left leg over the right knee. If you can't cross high in your legs, then cross low in your legs (shins or ankles). If you can, then tuck the left toes around our right calf. Don't force yourself into the position.

Bring your arms in front of you.

Take your left elbow and hook it underneath the right elbow.

Sit and hold for a couple of deep breaths. Feel the stretch.

Chair Pigeon Pose

Chair Kapotasana

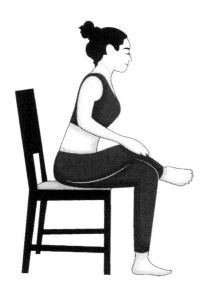

This pose helps open your hips, enhancing mobility and flexibility in the joint. In addition to stretching your hip flexors and lower back, pigeon pose alleviates mild lower back or hip pain by stretching these muscles regularly. A great way to ease lower back stiffness, with the focus on stretching the hamstrings and the gluteus.

Sit nice and tall, with your back straight.

Now inhale and raise the right leg, holding it carefully with your hands and place it over the left thigh, sitting comfortably.

In this chair pigeon pose, the flexing of the hip joint and the knee plays a role to keep them fit and flexible.

Once placed comfortably, sit straight if possible and take three breaths here, or as long as you need it. If bringing the leg over and placing it on the other is difficult, then lift the right leg and try and hold it in your arms for a few seconds and then slowly release. Repeat with the opposite side.

Chair Seated Twists

Chair Seated Twists are an effective exercise to stimulate the neck, hips and shoulders, while simultaneously engaging the muscles in one's back. The twisting action of the torso onto a grounded sit bone combined with regular practice helps to maintain mobility along one's spine. The chair provides excellent support, allowing one to easily remain in this twist while keeping their breath connected to their body movement. This practice can be used as a means of quickly releasing tension, energizing both body and mind.

Note: If you're recovering from surgery to your abdominal organs (like hernias, appendicitis, etc.), pelvic floor, or lower back (like a slipped disc), then this pose should be practiced after consulting a medical professional.

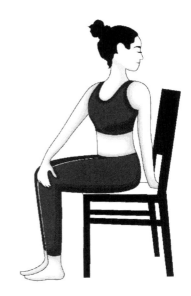

Listen to your body. Don't perform a twist pose if your body feels uncomfortable, tense, or in pain. Take extra care when performing any twist poses.

Sit comfortably on the chair with shoulders relaxed. Make sure you're not leaning onto the back of the chair. Rock forward and back, and feel your sit bones. Sit tall with feet touching the floor; knees hip-width apart.

Inhale and place your arms over your head—lift and lengthen.

With the exhalation, twist left from the base of the spine. Your ribcage, shoulders, neck, and eyes go to the left, but the hips remain on the chair.

The right hand goes to the left knee, and the left hand is behind the left hip.

Breathe and feel the air filling up your body, and lengthen.

Exhale, continue to twist until you find your edge, and hold there. Check your knees to see if they're still in line with each other, that one is not ahead of the other.

Take a couple of deep breaths. Keep your shoulders away from the ears.

Standing Forward Bend Chair

Uttanasana Chair

Stand in tadasana, extending your legs and tightening your kneecaps. Reach up to the ceiling with palms facing forward, elongating your whole body, then exhale and bend forward from the waist while keeping your legs fully stretched but not

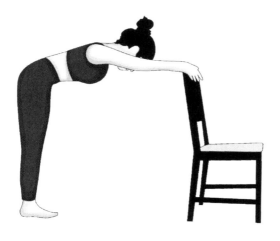

locked. Place both palms gently on a chair about three feet ahead of you and keep the length of your spine parallel to the floor as you push up through your sitting bones. Don't put your all weight on the chair. It's there to support you. Feel your abdominal muscles holding you and your back straight. Feel the energy radiating from the back of your legs and make sure that there is equal pressure on both the inner and outer edges of each foot. Stay in this pose for thirty to sixty seconds before releasing, repeating and trying to hold for longer if possible. As always, continue to breathe evenly throughout the practice.

Achy Joint Sequence

Chair Mountain Pose

Tadasana

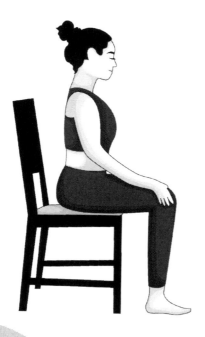

Despite being a primary seated position that could also be performed standing, tadasana has many benefits. This is one of the foundational poses (asanas) in yoga, the same as diaphragmatic (deep or belly) breathing for breathing (pranayama) practice. Tadasana keeps your body actively aligned, which requires a certain level of body awareness.

Sit comfortably in the middle of the chair. Leave some space between the back of the chair and your back. Rock forward and back to find the sit bones. Feet flat on the floor, hip-distance apart. If you prefer, bring your knees together.

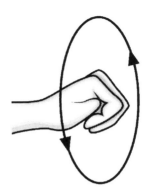

Start connecting to your breath.

Keep sitting in Tadasana pose. You can lean into your backrest if you want to. Still keep your knees at the square angle.

Start doing wrist rotations

One side and then another.

Repeat five to ten times on one side of each hand. You can rotate both wrists simultaneously or alternate them if you wish. Rotate them mindfully. Let the move be thoughtful.

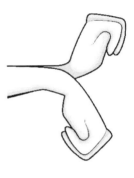

Ad wrist joint flexing, flex them up and down. Simultaneously or alternate them, five to ten times each hand.

On the inhale, bend the elbows and bring the fingers to your shoulders. Exhale—repeat this motion, moving the fingers from the shoulder to the shoulder and then extending the arms back in front of you. Inhale and exhale—repeat this about ten times with each arm.

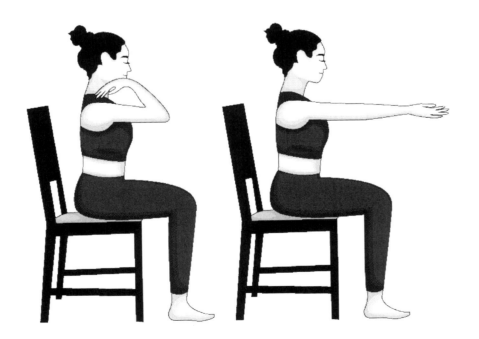

Wrist Flexion Stretch

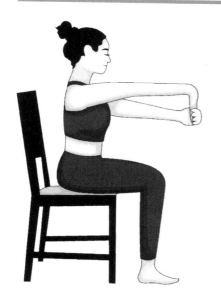

Inhale and extend your right arm straight out, palm facing down. Let your left hand take your right arms fingers and gently pull them towards your chest. You may feel a stretch on top of your forearm.

Stay here for three more breaths, gently going deeper into the stretch on each exhale while respecting your wrist's natural range of movement.

Stretch as far as you comfortably can without pain.

Then pull the fingers to the opposite side—fingers facing up.

Repeat the same to your left arm.

Shoulders Lift And Drop

Our joints store a lot of stress and tension. While it is easy to act normal as we watch TV, read, and perform our daily activities, we are involuntarily creating many blocks around them. This emotional stress is loaded with a lot of pain and tension around the joints. By doing these shoulder lifts with mindful breathing, you can ease a lot of tension points.

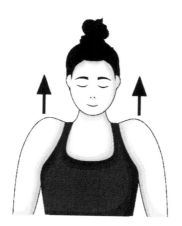
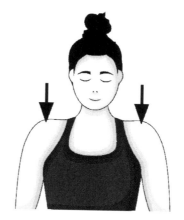

Sitting up tall and straight. Begin moving shoulders up as if you were trying to reach your earlobes. Inhale to raise the shoulders and exhale to drop the shoulders down.

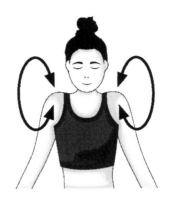

Mindfully do this coordinating movement with your ocean breath—five to eight times.

Carry on with shoulder rolls. Repeat five times to one side, and then to the opposite.

Goddess Pose on Chair

Utkata Konasana

This pose can be held longer given that the hips and sit bones are supported and remain stable.

It lengthens the spine by engaging the quadriceps, gluteus, hip flexors, inner thighs, and the joints of the hips, knees, and feet when the arms are raised up.

Sit nice and tall in the middle of the chair, leaving some room between your back and the backrest. Pressing through sits bones, open legs wide. Knees remain over ankles, and toes turn out slightly. Feel as if you're grounding through all four corners of your feet.

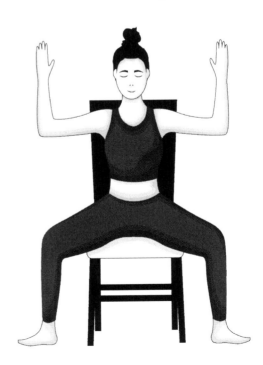

Feel the spine lengthen and keep an upright posture.

Extend arms and bend at the elbows with palms facing forward—cactus pose.

Squeeze your shoulder blades together slightly.

Lift chest up and outward. Feel the shoulder blades engage and the heart open.

To stay active in this pose, gently press through your heels and squeeze your shoulder blades.

Repeat for a couple of cycles of breath; lower your arms and repeat another three times.

Seated Forward Bend Pose Chair

Paschimottanasana

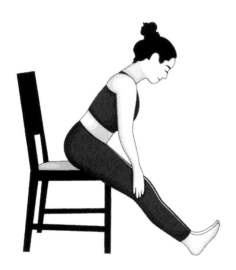

The pose is a great stretch for the lower back and hamstrings.

Note: People experiencing lower back or hamstring injuries should take this practice slowly.

Sit safely closer to the edge of your chair. Bring your legs out straight in front of you. Place your heels on the ground with your toes pointing out.

Breathe in, and check if your spine is straight. Lift your heart towards the sky.

Bend forward from the hips, keeping the spine elongated, but don't round it on your exhale. Keep legs straight but don't lock the knees. Have them slightly bent. If you need to bend them more, just do it. Listen to your body. Your arms can hang at your sides or you can put them on your legs but don't lean into them.

Hold for five breaths.

Feel how your hamstrings are stretching. If you need your hamstrings to stretch more, then pull your toes towards you.

Ankle Alphabet

Start from the mountain pose with your feet touching the floor.

Straighten your right leg in front of you with your toes pointing forward.

Extend your left leg with your toes pointed toward the ceiling. Imagine that you're using your big toe to write alphabet letters.

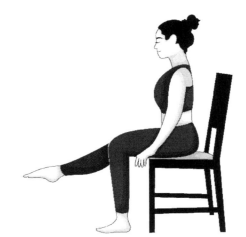

Lift your leg slightly from the floor and draw the letters twice. Repeat with the other leg.

Repeat twice, then switch to your other leg.

Once you're done, return to tadasana.

Sit nice and tall in mountain pose.

Lift your left foot and place it on the right thigh.

Stretch your big toe up and down and to the side with your fingers. Do it ten times and all different directions and then switch the foot.

Chair Mountain Pose Heel Raised

Sit nice and tall. Keep your shoulders relaxed. Your neck is nice and tall. Your arms can rest on your thighs. Take a few deep breaths. Check how you feel. Inhale and lift your one heel up or both. Take a couple deep breaths. Lower on the exhale, repeat with the other foot.

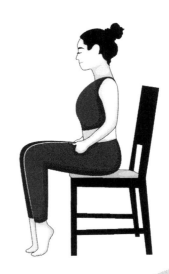

Repeat five times for each foot and remember to coordinate it with a breath.

Chair Flexing Foot Pose

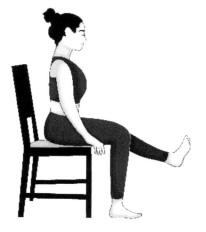

The Chair Flexing Foot Pose is a safe practice for students who have worn and torn ligaments at the knees and ankles, are healing from Achilles tendonitis, or are recovering from leg injuries or surgeries. A variation of this pose can also be performed lying in bed. During this movement, nerve cells in the joints are activated, resulting in better joint mobility and a better range of motion. This makes one's day-to-day activities easier to complete.

Draw the crown of your head towards the sky and lengthen your spine. Place your hands gently on your knees.

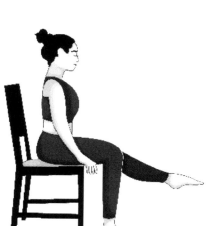

Begin by lifting the right leg and pointing the toes away from you.

Inhale, lift your toes towards your face, and press the heel away.

Exhale and point out the toes. Repeat a couple of rounds before switching the legs.

Repeat on the left side.

Repeat each leg four to six times.

This is a great movement to increase blood flow to the lower extremities of the body, which can aid in reducing leg lymphedema, varicose veins, and other possible discomforts in the calves and feet.

Sit and Stand

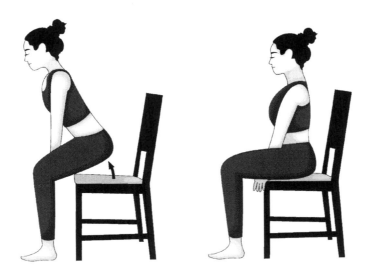

Sit nice and tall. Keep your shoulders relaxed. Your neck is nice and tall.

Slowly stand up and sit back down without using your arms for support. The movement should be slow and controlled. Repeat until you can't do it anymore. Rest for a minute, then repeat two times. If the chair is too low, start by rising from a cushion on the seat and removing it when you are finished.

Seated Forward Fold Pose on Chair

Forward fold can quickly release tensions in the upper body and helps to open the lower back, shoulders, neck, and hips. It aids in removing the tightness and stiffness of the muscles. It's a quick way to awaken and open the upper body joints, nerves, and muscles. The forward fold will help stretch the lower back and the entire spine.

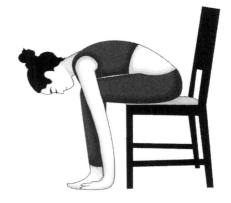

Note: If you have high blood pressure or difficulty breathing, you should not do this pose.

While seated in chair tadasana (mountain pose chair), breathe in deep a few times to relax and extend the spine. Exhaling, bring your arms down towards your feet, with the torso resting on the thighs and chin close to the knees. Stretching the shoulders, place your palms flat on the floor and remain here for four breaths. As you exhale, push closer into the thighs and abdomen, stretching farther each time. To release, inhale, look up first, then raise your arms before coming back to sit in chair tadasana. Repeat this process as needed for a longer duration. Use a cushion under your chest and diaphragm for extra support if you need it.

Headaches, Migraines and Neck Tension Relief Sequence

Chair Mountain Pose

Chair Tadasana

Sit comfortably in the middle of the chair. Leave some space between the back of the chair and your back.

Rock forward and back to find the sit bones.

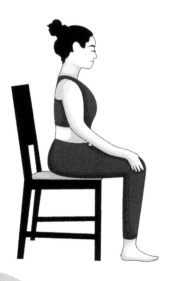

Feet flat on the floor, hip-distance apart. Feel your feet and floor connection. If you prefer, bring your knees together. Start drawing energy from the ground through your heels and legs.

Stack your head over your heart and heart over your pelvis.

Start connecting to your breath.

Take a couple of deep breaths.

Sit straight but with no tension in your body. Check that you are not hunching, that your neck feels long, the shoulders are resting, the chin is slightly tucked in.

Breathe in and out. Connect to your deep breath. Feel your rib cage and belly expanding. Slowly breathe it out.

Repeat for a couple of rounds.

Chair Neck Rolls

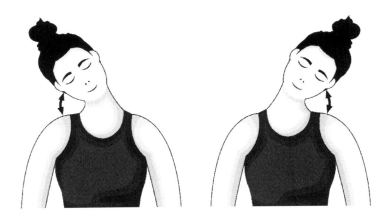

Chair neck rolls help to strengthen the neck, shoulders, and upper back.

People recovering from an accident, injury, or surgery could benefit from practicing roll necks, which can speed up the recovery. Extending, bending and rotating the neck regularly can help maintain a normal range of motion. Chair neck rolls are targeted at the joint called atlas just below the skull that uses deep neck flexor muscles to facilitate movement and reduce tension.

These movements can work wonders on the nervous system when coordinated with breathing.

Sit tall and straight with your head stacked over your heart and your heart over your hips. Feel your feet firmly placed on the ground, hip-distance apart. Leave some space between your and the chair's back.

Rest your arms on the knees or thighs with palms facing up or down.

Take a couple of deep breaths.

Inhale and move your ear towards the right shoulder and exhale.

On the inhale, come back to the center, exhale, and pause before switching sides.

Repeat on another side: inhale, move your ear towards the left shoulder, relax, and exhale. Then inhale and return to the center.

Note: keep your shoulders relaxed, don't try to lift your shoulders to the ear. You bend your neck as far as your body allows today. With practice, your body's flexibility will improve. Concentrate on coordinating your movement with breath rather than how far you can reach.

Repeat this movement from neck/ear to shoulders while coordinating breath and movement. You can close your eyes if you like, and keep the body still yet relaxed.

Return to the center and pause with your breath before moving on to the next neck movement. Repeat the movement three to five times on each side.

Remember to breathe deeply.

Neck U Rotation Close Up

Kantha U Paryaayakrama

This stretches and strengthens the muscles around the neck and shoulders and the muscles in the upper back. The twist strengthens the side of the neck.

While the movement may seem simple, the improved range of motion helps with other poses and day-to-day activities.

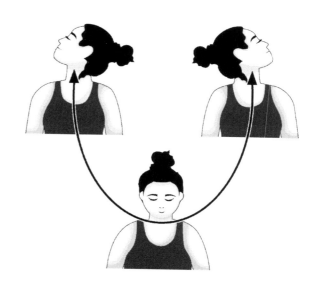

Note: Avoid this pose if you have had any recent injury or surgery to the neck, shoulders, or upper back. Also, if you have acute spondylitis and extreme pain in the neck and shoulders or are experiencing an eye or ear infection, severe headache, migraine, vertigo, or dizziness, you should avoid this pose too.

Sit comfortably in the chair with a straight spine and feet on the floor. Let your arms rest at your sides. As you inhale, turn your head to the left, exhale, and tuck your chin towards your chest. Inhaling once more, move your chin toward the right shoulder, and exhale, rolling it back to your chest. Alternate between both sides until you return to a neutral position with the chin parallel to the floor.

Stay here for three rounds.

Chair Cat-Cow Pose

Chair Marjaryasana Bitilasana

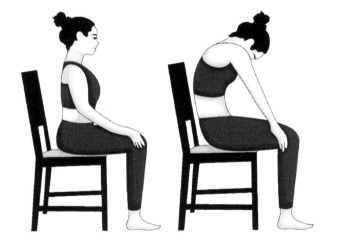

Chair cat-cow pose is an effective way to tackle back pain and neck and shoulder stiffness. This therapeutic practice boosts flexibility as it stretches and massages the abdominal cavity, helping to improve digestion. Additionally, it increases the oxygenated blood supply in the spine, allowing a smoother and less painful movement of the back and neck muscles. Those with rheumatoid arthritis or osteoarthritis can benefit from this pose as the regular practice may help prevent these conditions from developing and reduce their symptoms at early stages.

Note: If you have a neck injury, shoulder, spine, or hip injury, or have had recent abdominal surgery, you should avoid practicing the cat-cow pose until you check with your doctor first.

Also, please **do not round** your spine if you have osteopenia or osteoporosis. On your exhale—return to a **neutral spine** instead of rounding.

Sit in a mountain pose. Relax and connect to your breath. Sit up tall. Feel the crown of your head rising towards the ceiling. Connect to your breath and take a couple of deep breaths. Rest your feet on the floor and keep your knees aligned with your hips.

Put your arms on your knees.

On the inhale, expand your chest. Let your head and chin go slightly back.

On the exhale, round your spine by curling the chest in.

Check that your shoulders are relaxed. Feel the space between your shoulders and earlobes. Keep breathing.

Practice coordinating your breath with the movement. Don't rush. Smile, inhale, and repeat the movement—three to five times.

Chair Seated Side Stretch Pose

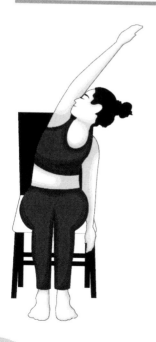

This pose opens the shoulders and the neck. The arms are stretched to the opposite way. It is a great way to stretch for people with knee injuries. In addition to stretching, you increase awareness of your diaphragm and breathing.

Sit upright and keep knees hip-width apart or together. Place the hands on either side of the seat or your lap.

Roll your shoulders down the back.

Inhale pulling in the core, sweep the right arm above the head, creating a lateral bend on the left-hand side. Exhale into the stretch. Allow your chest and head to tilt to the left. Stay in this pose for three breaths.

On the inhale, return to the center.

Repeat the same with the left side.

You can choose to stay on one side for two to three breaths before switching to the other side, or you may choose to move dynamically between one side and the other on the breath. Do what feels best for your body. During the movement, you may look down at the floor, straight ahead or up towards the top arm—please choose the option that feels right for your neck. Try to keep your mouth and jaw loose as you move.

Chair Seated Twists

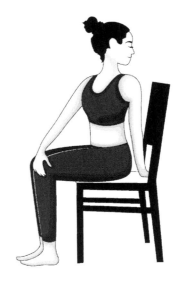

Chair seated twist is an effective exercise to stimulate the neck, hips and shoulders, while simultaneously engaging the muscles in one's back. The twisting action of the torso onto a grounded sit bone, combined with regular practice, helps to maintain mobility along one's spine. The chair provides excellent support, allowing one to easily remain in this twist while keeping their breath connected to their body movement. This practice can be used as a means of quickly releasing tension, energizing both body and mind.

Note: If you're recovering after surgery to abdominal organs (like hernias, appendicitis, etc.), the pelvic floor, or lower back (like a slipped disc), you should consult a medical professional before practicing this pose.

Listen to your body. Don't perform a twist pose if your body feels uncomfortable, tense, or in pain. Take extra care when performing any twist poses.

Sit comfortably on the chair with shoulders relaxed.

Make sure you're not leaning onto the back of the chair. Rock forward and back, find your sit bones. Sit tall with feet touching the floor; knees hip-width apart.

Inhale and place your arms over your head—lift and lengthen.

With the exhalation, twist left from the base of the spine. Your ribcage, shoulders, neck, and eyes go to the left, but the hips remain on the chair.

The right hand goes to the left knee, and the left hand is behind the left hip or on the back of the chair.

Breathe and feel the air filling up your body, and lengthen.

Eagle Arms

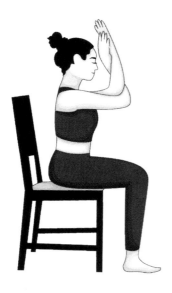

The whole back muscles are stretched, so it's a quick way to relieve shoulder and neck stiffness.

Sit comfortably on a chair, back straight, and feet firmly grounded on the floor. Take a few breaths here.

Cross the elbows, taking the right over left.

Interlock the arms. Bring your mind to the breath and stay for three breaths.

Release and repeat on the opposite side. Take and cross your left elbow over the right. Keep breathing for another three breaths. Release. Come back to the center.

Cobra Pose Chair

Bhujangasana

This pose strengthens your legs, upper back, lower back, shoulders, hamstrings, hips, glutes, and feet by engaging your legs, upper back, lower back, shoulders, hamstrings, hips, glutes, and feet. It can also help relieve stiffness in your shoulders, back, arms, and legs and elongate and lengthen your back.

Sit up nice and tall, closer to the edge of the chair, with your shoulders relaxed. Keep your knees together or hips apart.

Open your chest. Squeeze your shoulder blades together, look up, and bring your hands to the back of the chair.

Take the arms behind you on the inhale and hold on to the chair. Raise the chest and shoulders to look up. Your chin tilts upward and your eyes gaze toward the heavens.

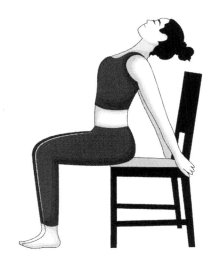

Exhale, stay here in cobra pose chair feeling the stretch at the neck and upper chest.

Smile as you remain here for six breaths, breathing slow and deep. With each exhalation, feel the stretch.

Release, relax, and repeat, staying for the second round of six breaths.

Seated Forward Fold Pose on Chair

Forward fold can quickly release tensions in the upper body and help to open the lower back, shoulders, neck, and hips. It aids in removing the tightness and stiffness of the muscles. A quick way to awaken and open the upper body joints, nerves, and muscles. The forward fold will help stretch the lower back and the entire spine.

Note: If you have high blood pressure or difficulty breathing, you should not do this pose.

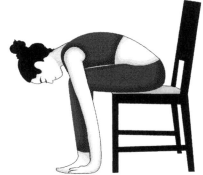

While seated in chair tadasana (mountain pose chair), breathe in deep a few times to relax and extend the spine. Exhaling, bring your arms down towards your feet, with the torso resting on the thighs and chin close to the knees. Stretching the shoulders, place your palms flat on the floor and remain here for four breaths. As you exhale, push closer into the thighs and abdomen, stretching farther each time. To release, inhale, look up first, then raise your arms before coming back to sit in chair tadasana. Repeat this process as needed for a longer duration. Use a cushion under your chest and diaphragm for extra support if you need it.

Conclusion

Now you have all the tools to reach for the sky while sitting down. You are equipped with the knowledge to improve your mental health and focus, your physical strength and flexibility, and your mindfulness. No matter what the reason may be that you are forced to "stay down," you can now reach for greater heights with confidence and with stillness of mind and soul.

I hope this book has proved to you that your mobility, your age, your flexibility, your physical health, your balance, etc., do not have the ability to hold you back from wellness or living a mindful lifestyle. There is nothing holding you back. You can do this.

You Could Be Key to Someone Else's Yoga Journey

Now that you're ready to reap all the benefits chair yoga has to offer, you have a unique opportunity to help someone else.

Simply by sharing your honest opinion of this book on Amazon, you'll show other readers that they can benefit too – and exactly where they can find the guidance they need to make sure they do.

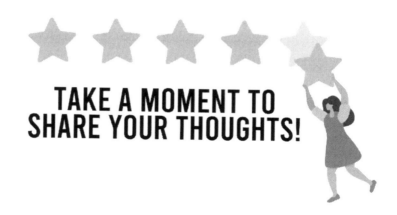

TAKE A MOMENT TO SHARE YOUR THOUGHTS!

Thank you so much for your support. No matter what might hold us back from standing yoga, we can still access its astounding potential... And with your help, I can make sure that the message reaches even more people.

References

8 yoga myths to stop believing today. (2019, June 21). Cleveland Clinic. https://health.clevelandclinic.org/think-you-cant-do-yoga-you-might-be-believing-one-of-these-8-yoga-myths/

Anne, H. (2019, June 17). 7 reasons why warmup and proper breathing is important for yoga. Simplejoy.co.uk. https://simplejoy.co.uk/2019/06/17/warmup-and-breathing-in-yoga/

Better Health Channel. (2012). Ageing - muscles bones and joints. Vic.gov.au. https://www.betterhealth.vic.gov.au/health/conditionsandtreatments/ageing-muscles-bones-and-joints

Bisht, H. (2022, September 28). Benefits of bhramari pranayama and how to do it. PharmEasy Blog. https://pharmeasy.in/blog/health-fitness-benefits-of-bhramari-pranayama-and-how-to-do-it/

Burgin, T. (2012, May 11). Dirga pranayama. Yoga Basics. https://www.yogabasics.com/practice/dirga-pranayama/

Burgin, T. (2021, June 8). Sama vritti pranayama (box breath or equal breathing). Yoga Basics. https://www.yogabasics.com/practice/sama-vritti-pranayama/

Chalicha, E. (2022, November 8). Should You Do Chair Yoga Every Day? BetterMe Blog. https://betterme.world/articles/chair-yoga-every-day

Cronkleton, E. (2018, August 15). How to breathe and ways to breathe better. Healthline. https://www.healthline.com/health/how-to-breathe#stronger-diaphragm

Excellence in Fitness. (n.d.). How long does it take for older adults to build muscle? Excellence in Fitness. Retrieved February 10, 2023, from https://www.excellenceinfitness.com/blog/how-long-does-it-take-for-older-adults-to-build-muscle

Guillemets, T. (2002). Yoga quotes (hatha yoga, asanas, etc.). Www.quotegarden.com. https://www.quotegarden.com/yoga.html

Instafitness. (2019, March 13). 9 popular types of yoga- modern yoga styles you should try. Instafitness. https://instafitness.in/9-popular-yoga-types/

J, S. (2022, May 3). The evolution of yoga over time. Mind Is the Master. https://mindisthemaster.com/evolution-of-yoga-over-time/

Lakshmi Voelker Chair Yoga. (n.d.). Chair yoga faqs. LV Chair Yoga. Retrieved February 9, 2023, from https://www.lvchairyoga.com/chair-yoga-faqs

LifeStyle Desk. (2022, November 28). Top 5 reasons you should make yoga warmup part of your workout. News18. https://www.news18.com/news/lifestyle/top-5-reasons-you-should-make-yoga-warmup-part-of-your-workout-6491773.html

Living Maples. (2022, July 2). Chair yoga for seniors, beginner friendly. Living Maples. https://livingmaples.com/mag/chair-yoga-for-seniors

Mandala Yoga. (2020, April 15). How did yoga evolve into what we practice today? Mandala Yoga. https://mandalayoga.ie/evolution_of_yoga/

McGee, K. (2017, February 27). Chair yoga warm-ups: Poses to get your blood flowing. Kristin McGee. https://kristinmcgee.com/chair-yoga-warm-ups

MPH, C. A., MD, & MD, N. R. (2021, December 6). Yoga for weight loss: Benefits beyond burning calories. Harvard Health. https://www.health.harvard.edu/blog/yoga-for-weight-loss-benefits-beyond-burning-calories-202112062650

Newlyn, E. (2016). The 8 limbs of yoga explained. Ekhartyoga.com. https://www.ekhartyoga.com/articles/philosophy/the-8-limbs-of-yoga-explained

Newlyn, E. (2017, October 9). What is hatha yoga? Ekhart Yoga. https://www.ekhartyoga.com/articles/philosophy/what-is-hatha-yoga

Nunez, K. (2020, May 15). Pranayama benefits for physical and emotional health. Healthline. https://www.healthline.com/health/pranayama-benefits#less-stress

OriGym. (2022, March 8). History of yoga: Origins to modern day. OriGym. https://origympersonaltrainercourses.co.uk/blog/history-of-yoga#where

Pat's Chair Yoga. (n.d.). FAQs. Pat's Chair Yoga. Retrieved February 10, 2023, from https://patschairyoga.com/faqs/

Pizer, A. (2020a, June 3). Step by step instructions for dirga pranayama three-part breath. Verywell Fit. https://www.verywellfit.com/three-part-breath-dirga-pranayama-3566762

Pizer, A. (2020b, June 30). Easily learn ujjayi breath to deepen your yoga practice. Verywell Fit. https://www.verywellfit.com/ocean-breath-ujjayi-pranayama-3566763

Senior Lifestyle. (2020, February 12). Top 10 chair yoga positions for seniors [infographic]. Senior Lifestyle. https://www.seniorlifestyle.com/resources/blog/infographic-top-10-chair-yoga-positions-for-seniors

ShareCare. (n.d.). What is the difference between traditional and contemporary yoga? | yoga. Sharecare. Retrieved February 10, 2023, from https://www.sharecare.com/health/yoga/what-difference-traditional-contemporary-yoga

Singleton, M. (2011, February 4). The origins of yoga: Ancient + modern philosophies of the practice. Yoga Journal. https://www.yogajournal.com/yoga-101/philosophy/yoga-s-greater-truth/

Smith, L. (2023, February 23). 45 of the best yoga quotes to motivate, uplift and inspire you. The Good Body. https://www.thegoodbody.com/yoga-quotes/

Stump, M. (2017, June 16). Yoga and its many benefits. Lifespan. https://www.lifespan.org/lifespan-living/yoga-and-its-many-benefits

University of Michigan Health. (n.d.). Diaphragmatic breathing for GI patients. Www.uofmhealth.org. https://www.uofmhealth.org/conditions-treatments/digestive-and-liver-health/diaphragmatic-breathing-gi-patients

WebMD. (2021, October 25). What to know about alternate-nostril breathing. WebMD. https://www.webmd.com/balance/what-to-know-about-alternate-nostril-breathing

Wu, Y., Johnson, B. T., Acabchuk, R. L., Chen, S., Lewis, H. K., Livingston, J., Park, C. L., & Pescatello, L. S. (2019). Yoga as antihypertensive lifestyle therapy: A systematic review and meta-analysis. Mayo Clinic Proceedings, 94(3). https://doi.org/10.1016/j.mayocp.2018.09.023

Zerbe, L. (2021, April 21). Use this gentle chair yoga for seniors routine to reduce pain & anxiety. Dr. Axe. https://draxe.com/fitness/chair-yoga-for-seniors/

Made in the USA
Monee, IL
24 October 2023

45125177R00083